Affirmations,
Meditations,
and
Encouragements
for
Women Living
with
Breast Cancer

Affirmations, Meditations, and Encouragements for Women Living with Breast Cancer

LINDA DACKMAN

HarperSanFrancisco
A Division of HarperCollins*Publishers*

For Willa, Peggy, and Jane,
and all the other women, too numerous to mention.

AFFIRMATIONS, MEDITATIONS, AND ENCOURAGEMENTS
FOR WOMEN LIVING WITH BREAST CANCER. Copyright
© 1991 by Linda Dackman. All rights reserved. Printed in
the United States of America. No part of this book may be
used or reproduced in any manner whatsoever without
written permission except in the case of brief quotations em-
bodied in critical articles and reviews. For information ad-
dress HarperCollins Publishers, 10 East 53rd Street, New
York, NY 10022.
Reprinted by arrangement with Lowell House, a division
of RGA Publishing Group, Inc.

FIRST HARPERCOLLINS PAPERBACK EDITION
PUBLISHED IN 1992

Library of Congress Cataloging-in-Publication Data
Dackman, Linda.
    Affirmations, meditations, and encouragements for
women living with breast cancer / Linda Dackman.
        p. cm.
    Originally published: Los Angeles : Lowell House,
1991.
    Includes index.
    1.Breast—Cancer—Psychological aspects.
    2. Meditations. I. Title.
    RC280.B6D32 1993   92-53907
    362.1'9699449-dc20   CIP

92 93 94 95 96 ❖ HAD 10 9 8 7 6 5 4 3 2 1

This edition is printed on acid-free paper that meets the
American National Standards Institute Z39.48 Standard.

Table of Contents

Introduction   1

After Diagnosis   5

Decision Making   21

Surgery   43

Coping with Radiation and Chemotherapy   67

Body and Self   105

Reconstruction   129

Relationships   155

Concerns of Single Women   179

Sexuality   207

Sex and Nudity   235

Transformations   255

Index   281

Introduction

I was a young single woman when I was diagnosed with breast cancer in 1985 at the age of thirty-four. I had no psychological preparation for what the doctors discovered on my right breast during a routine exam; there was no known family history and there had been no worrisome lump. As had millions of women before me, I went through the terror and the fear, the juggling of opinions, the loss of my breast, the living with uncertainty, and the psychological struggles of returning to life without all the equipment to play the game.

I was so shaken by my experience with breast cancer that I resolved to become a Reach to Recovery volunteer the following year. Since 1986 I have counseled countless women as they find themselves newly faced with this disease. I also began writing about my experience. I published an article about breast cancer in *Vogue* magazine, as well as a book, *Up Front,* about the physical and psychological recovery from breast cancer.

As a result of my experience in writing and speaking about breast cancer from the patient's point of view, I was asked to write this book, *Affirmations, Meditations, and Encouragements for Women Living with Breast Cancer.* Down-to-earth, yet inspiring, this book includes the voices of many women, including myself, who have been confronted with breast cancer. It is the sum total of many perspectives, experiences, and voices, interwoven and laid out one upon the other.

The scope ranges from the first shock of diagnosis to the ultimately transformative powers of the breast cancer experience—and most of the joys and fears in between. You might say that this volume is like a breast cancer support group between the covers of a book: it is exactly what a woman recuperating in her hospital bed or at any of the other milestones of treatment and recovery might need—the accumulated coping devices, black humor, wisdom, and experiences of other women who have preceded her in living with breast cancer.

Affirmations, Meditations, and Encouragements offers all sorts of moments, taken randomly or consecutively, that together describe the arduous journey through a first diagnosis with breast cancer. Gathered here are moving, funny, poignant anecdotes and practical information, of value to every woman concerned with or diagnosed with this disease.

Affirmations, Meditations, and Encouragements is built upon the experiences of women of all ages, ranging from twenty-three to seventy; women who have undergone all types of breast surgery and treatments from lumpectomy and mastectomy to radiation and chemotherapy; women who are married, single, divorced, widowed; and in the appropriate chapters, the perspectives of their partners.

Since a confrontation with breast cancer is an intense and extraordinary period in a woman's life, this book is not keyed to the days of the year like the usual daily meditation book. Instead, each page stands whole and distinct on its own, as well as being loosely grouped into chapters that correspond to the progress of a woman's experience.

Approach this book as you like. Read through it in sequence, moving from diagnosis on to surgery and chemotherapy and the many other physical, psychological, and emotional aftermaths of breast cancer, or read and reread at random, based on your own daily shifting questions, concerns, and needs. In either case, you will touch on topics as universal as fear and terror and as intimate as sexual shame. Some pages are descriptions or summations. Some are the experiences of women, as varied and creative in their wisdom, weaknesses, and strategies as the individuals who offer them. Each page ends with an affirmation, meditation, or encouragement that you may use as a tool in your recovery.

My hope is that you find this book to be inspirational, uplifting, and practical. It is a place for you to uncover, for example, what it means to be "in the chemo" or to wring out a wet prosthesis, and to cry and laugh out loud at the ways in which others have managed to cope. It is a place for you to share others' experiences and to gain new insights. But most important, this book is a private place for you to feel supported and understood, a place to somehow share your grief, anger, and sense of loss. Above all, it is a resource to strengthen you in your journey of self-discovery and newly deepened appreciation of life.

After Diagnosis

Courage is very important. Like a muscle,
it is strengthened by use.
—*Ruth Gordon*

∼

What follows a breast cancer diagnosis? Shock. Horror.
Disbelief. Fear. Panic. Terror.

The question, "Cancer?"

The answer, "Yes, cancer!"

And then what?

Then you just go on.

I strengthen my courage just by going on.

The time on either side of *now* stands fast.
—*Maxine Kumin*

~

Despite our fears and suspicions, hearing the actual diagnosis of breast cancer from a doctor is always a shock. And in its wake, time stands still.

As Jory Graham points out in her book, *In the Company of Others,* what you hear in those first few stony seconds as time grinds to a halt is "less like a medical fact from a doctor and more like a verdict from a judge. What you hear is 'I have been sentenced to death,' and in your heart of hearts you know that it is for a crime that you did not commit."

Ms. Graham's metaphor is apt. All you have to remember is that there is no judge and that you are the prosecution, the defense, and the jury.

I acknowledge that the diagnosis of cancer is a terrible shock, but a diagnosis alone does not condemn me.

It is by surmounting difficulties, not by sinking
under them, that we discover our fortitude.

—*Hannah Webster Foster*

∽

Who can know what might have been different if your
physical problem had been dealt with sooner? Feel your
anger. Grieve for the delay. But, more important, get angry
about the diagnosis of cancer itself. This is the time to ask,
what can I do about it now? Self-pity changes nothing.
Take your anger and use it positively. Let it spur you on to
the next step, which is the fighting.

*No matter how painful the circumstances of when and how I
heard the news, now is the time to fight against
breast cancer. Starting today, I fight.*

Shock

Though the body moves, the soul may stay behind.
—*Murasaki Shikibu*

The world moves; our bodies move; but time and our souls stand still. Our minds rush off without us, to visit some distant, very narrow place at the end of a long, dark tunnel. Without looking into it, we understand that place, although our thoughts cannot stay there long.

Then, for a moment or two, we return to the world as we once knew it. We cannot understand why it hasn't changed. All that has changed is our own world. We have taken the word *cancer* inside us, and everything else is shattered.

Despite my shock and disorientation, I continue.

I'm so angry that my body's
all but bursting into flame.

—*Alamanda*

~

The anger we feel is terrifying, directed as it is against the very universe. The anger within us erupts, sudden, wrenching, seemingly irrevocable, and we scream, "How dare this happen to me?" We are raging against the implication that our lives as we have known them are about to be destroyed. We are burning with anger at the threat to our plans, our expectations, our ideas about the future.

Think of this anger as an erupting volcano, because from the volcano—as from anger—also come renewal and rebirth. As the earth gives birth to itself by erupting, we can think of ourselves as self-renewing by channeling anger, fear, and pain about this diagnosis into creative action and the vital will to fight.

My anger is a tool in the fight against this disease.

Rage

. . . Do the hardest thing on earth for you. . . .
—Katherine Mansfield

≈

Do the hardest thing on earth for you, spew out your rage. Sit with it. Find it. Feel it. Talk it out with yourself. Stamp your feet. Cry. Punch pillows. Let the child in you begin to rage against the unfairness of this news. "Me? How could I have cancer?" Park your car in a secluded spot and scream. "Get out. Get out!" Scream into roaring waves, or from a hilltop, or in the shadow and the din of a passing train. Rage against cancer by screaming it out. Because suddenly, to swallow rage or deny it feels too much like poison. Send it out, spew it out, shout it out.

Today I shout, "Get out, get out, get ooouuuuttt!"
to cancer and to my rage.

... Terrors ... all derive their dread sublimity from Death.
—*Susan Edmonstone Ferrier*

◇

Terror wells up from some place deep within the body and soul, bypassing the conscious mind completely. We tremble uncontrollably in it, as it goes beyond feeling to being. It is "being terror," and the terror is the fear and the pain of death.

Even in the middle of it, we are somehow aware of how totally at one with terror we are. And that is how, while we are lost in its utter sharpness, we also manage to bring ourselves back from its jagged edge. Gradually, awareness returns. We know we have just confronted the terror of death, and having done so, we are even more certain that we want to survive.

The experience of terror galvanizes my will to fight.

Grief

I tell you hopeless grief is passionless.
—*Elizabeth Barrett Browning*

∾

I have breast cancer, you say to yourself over and over again
—yet you do not fully grasp the meaning of these words.
The impact approaches and then recedes, comes to you
painfully clear, then muffled, then spoken in a foreign language that you simply cannot understand. You are inside and
outside yourself all at once, aware that something awful has
happened but at the same time expecting to wake up from
this terrible dream. You are rocked by shock and fear and
grief. Then suddenly you shift, you are above it all, floating calmly, looking down at the world. Then you can't
help but notice the shattered pieces of yourself on the floor.
Finally, you scream and cry.

*I do not fear the passion of my grief because in the long run
its energy propels me forward.*

Oh Lord! If you but knew what a brimstone of a creature
I am behind all this beautiful amiability!

—*Jane Welsh Carlyle*

No matter how calm you may appear on the surface, you
are dancing on unstable ground. No one can absorb the
news of breast cancer simply by hearing the words that im-
part the diagnosis. The overwhelming reality of it becomes
instantly buried. But like the molten lava beneath the earth's
surface, it bubbles up from beneath the protective shell of
shock that surrounds you until you are ready to face it again.
To be in control and well organized is one common reaction. But remember that no matter how together you appear, even to yourself, you want to also respect and
acknowledge the chaos beneath.

*I acknowledge that under the surface all is chaos, and I trust
that when I face it again, I can handle it.*

It seems that the best armor is the rational mind.
—*Sarah J. McCarthy*

∼

Working through means capturing our experiences, feelings, hopes, and fears by crying, getting angry, shouting, thinking, meditating, writing, organizing, and talking to others, all in order to begin to define and understand our experience. With the shock of breast cancer, we must go through it over and over and over again. We talk, cry, scream, swear repeatedly because that is how we take hold, work through, and begin to master our fear and prepare ourselves for future treatment.

I use all the tools at my disposal to work through my feelings of fear and shock about this disease.

To be alone is to be different, to be different is to be alone.
—*Suzanne Gordon*

Who around you can really understand? Do they have cancer? Are they suddenly facing death? What do they know? You ask yourself these questions because you have the feeling of being cut off from people who haven't had to face this experience, even your husband. Maybe he is a very supportive husband, a psychologist at that, a man whose own profession is empathy. Maybe you have worked and lived together every day for over 25 years, but it doesn't matter. Breast cancer has a surreal, distancing effect.

Thoughts and feelings of distance are natural. But while you are floating above the world and looking down, don't get caught in a place of isolation, stuck between the tragedy of your fate and bitterness over what the world has done to you.

*In my thoughts lies the wellspring of my own hope. I focus on
thoughts that bring me closer to other people and that
leave me an opening through which to reach.*

Self-Blame

I don't say she was above reproach. She was
just above self-reproach.
—*Helen Caldwell*

~

A friend visited and brought along her new baby. The
thought of this new life at the time of my own brush with
death hurt at first, until I began to see myself in that infant. I was feeling equally fragile, equally needing and de-
serving of endless love and attention. It became very clear
to me: An infant doesn't deserve blame for what happens
to it, and no matter what, it still needs comfort and love.
I wasn't an infant but I saw that I was equally innocent and
equally needing of comfort. In that instant I forgave myself
for what had happened to me. Suddenly, I knew I didn't
create the cancer inside me and I didn't deserve blame.

If I hold myself like a loving mother, I won't have a
free hand to point the finger of self-blame.

Control

~

My philosophy is to exercise control, and believe me, I have come at this with both barrels blasting. But I have also cried and screamed and devoted a lot of time to letting my feelings out.

I have let go in other ways as well. I have let go of outcomes because I am fully aware that I cannot control them. What I can control is myself. My point is that to cry and to let go are ways of mastering the emotional roller coaster which immediately follows a diagnosis. It is the other half of the definition of control and just as important as being tough, directed, and scrappy.

Today I broaden my definition of control to include weeping and letting go.

Loss of Self

I came to see the damage that was done and
the treasures that prevail.

—Adrienne Rich

∼

No matter who you are and how tough, encountering cancer awakens all kinds of fears, threats, and anxieties. It is a
threat to your life, to your integrity, to your sense of self,
and your identity as a woman.

All you can strive for is to bring the "I" you know yourself to be and the new "I," so recently defined by cancer,
together. Try to retain the knowledge of yourself as diagnosed with cancer, but without having it negate the self
you once knew yourself to be.

*My knowledge of cancer merges with everything else that I know
to be true about me, yet it never exclusively defines me.*

I am one of those people who just can't help getting a kick
out of life—even when it's a kick in the teeth.

—*Polly Adler*

∿

Strange as this sounds, I told myself that if I had to have
this disease, then I was *uniquely qualified* to have it. I am a
physician and I have faced death before. I have faced mor-
tality many times, even my own, and have made peace with
myself.

That isn't to say that there aren't problems. Once you
become a physician-patient, it is also harder. There is no
innocence.

That is why all women, physicians or not, might benefit by my attitude. Each of us is uniquely qualified to cope
in our own way. By looking inside, we find ways in which
we are especially physically and emotionally prepared for
what lies ahead. Each of us has something special to rely
on.

I am uniquely qualified to cope with this disease.

Decision Making

Indecision

> All [life] is pattern . . . but we can't always see
> the pattern when we're part of it.
> —*Belva Plain*

~

Have you ever sailed a boat? You can't go in a straight line because you are dependent on capturing the wind in your sail. So you tack back and forth, zigzagging across the imaginary straight line that leads to your port. Deciding about cancer treatment is like that, too.

Mastectomy? Lumpectomy and radiation? Segmental? Reconstruction? All you can do is sail back and forth on swells of emotion and doubt, propelled forward by the force of research. As in sailing, the back-and-forth motion of making up your mind is really the only way to get the wind behind you and get you where you want to go.

My decision is still in the process of becoming.

God made the world round so we would never
be able to see too far down the road.

—*Isak Dinesen*

You are doing the best you can in this process, at a pace you can handle. It is a fine balancing act, to gather information when each bit of information stimulates new worries and upsets the balance. The anxiety may become so intense as to temporarily cut off your desire to know. Be patient. Accept that as each piece of information hits home, it causes another shock wave. But as the disease becomes more real, it also becomes more manageable.

When the shock waves are too intense and you back off, congratulate yourself for being so practical. It is your mind's way of keeping you from looking too far down the road until such time as you recover your balance. Trust that there is an inner self that will ensure it gets the information it needs.

*I'll put my glasses back on tomorrow when I'm again
ready to see to the horizon.*

"I have arguments with myself."
   "About what?"
   "Between the part of me that believes in things, and the part that doesn't."
   "And which wins?"
   "Sometimes one. Sometimes the other."
   "Then stop arguing."

—*Penelope Mortimer*

I felt that the doctors gave me too much information. For me, I wanted it simple and basic. I didn't want all the choices. There was something about all the discussion that felt too negative. I'd rather just see things as half full. I know my point of view is not popular these days, but I know myself. I am highly suggestible, and so my solution was to control the flow of information. I recognize that I don't need a great deal of research in my decision making, so my self-affirmation was to find one doctor that I totally trusted.

Knowing myself, I know how much information
I really want or need.

Have you come to the Red Sea place in your life
Where, in spite of all you can do,
There is no way out, there is no way back,
There is no other way but through?

—*Annie Johnson Flint*

Acknowledge that your choices don't seem like choices to you. They are severely circumscribed, limited, and difficult. You are anxious . . . terrified. Scream that you wish life was otherwise, then face that it is not. No one is more aware than you of the painfulness of what lies ahead, and yet it is up to you to choose it. Think about the process of choosing. Hard as it is, doesn't having and making the choice render it less painful?

*I freely accept my choices for treatment. That I have
a choice to make satisfies me.*

The facts of the present won't sit still for a portrait. They are constantly vibrating, full of clutter and confusion.

—*Macneile Dixon*

Amid the questions and the answers there is confusion. The decision process is one of change, racing to make sense of so much so fast and constantly finding new doors to open and new questions and options to investigate and pursue. It feels so urgent, yet progress seems so slow. Think of the process as something that brings order to the chaos while you are in the middle of the chaos itself. Your research into treatment options brings back a sense of control over your life. And it ultimately controls another form of chaos—the growth of cells in your body.

I will carry a notebook in which to write down my questions. They are the first steps in the process of mastery, organization, and control.

Intuition is a spiritual faculty and does not explain,
but simply points the way.

—*Florence Scovel Shinn*

Listen to the facts. And trust your own gut feelings. There is logic, but feelings are equally important. Initiate a dialogue between head, heart, and stomach in assimilating all that you hear. Remember, too, that it is possible for gut feelings to change. Some women describe how they started their decision-making process with the absolute certainty that they would have a lumpectomy, for example. Some women adhere to their gut feeling even in the face of contrary medical opinions. Yet when they go back to their guts, they find out that mastectomy is the choice for them. Once you are informed, trust that you will know what is necessary and right for you.

My treatment decision comes from what I learn and from what I find inside. In other words, my treatment decision comes from me.

To understand everything makes one tolerant.
—*Germaine de Staël*

❧

Don't worry if anyone thinks you're a lunatic because you are going around interviewing doctors carrying a cassette recorder. A diagnosis of breast cancer is a crash course in the disease. There is technical information to digest at a time when stress makes information hard to hear and even harder to assimilate. I tossed in bed late at night, playing havoc with the rush of words I *thought* I remembered from my doctor. I played it over and over a million times in my head, and each time the picture got worse. One way to short-circuit those fears and insecurities is to document what you hear, exactly as it was said. Start carrying a recorder.

I do whatever I have to do to inform myself.

I'm the foe of moderation, the champion of excess. . . .
　　　　　　　—*Tallulah Bankhead*

～

The cancer experience, when we are right in the middle of it, does not always feel controllable. We are being told that the doctors will try this and then that. We trust that it is for our good, but there are times when that's not how it feels. At those moments, buck the system to get what you need.

Ask for first opinions or impressions while promising that you will not hold the doctor to it: "I know you need the corroboration of God and everyone else, but based on what you have seen, what do you think?"

Insist that you not have to wait until Monday for what you have every right to hear on Friday.

One woman was told by a doctor that her tumor was too small to test for estrogen receptors. She said thank you and found a doctor who said there was no problem running that test on so small a sample.

I've heard from one famous Beverly Hills oncologist that in his community, six medical opinions are the minimum standard. So anything up to six is not excessive, it's moderate!

I know how "for my own good" feels, and I know when
"my own good" feels satisfied.

She found out there was no doctor
for her like Dr. "Have-To."

—*Elizabeth Phelps*

~

As soon as I knew it was cancer, I wanted my breast off as soon as possible. I was very clear that it was nothing next to my life. Mourn that breast? That breast was awful. It had betrayed me. It was no longer my friend.

I am inherently in charge of myself. No one else can tell me how to resolve my problems or how to live.

> Where, after all, do universal human rights begin? In small
> places, close to home—so close and so small that they
> cannot be seen on any map of the world.
>
> —*Eleanor Roosevelt*

∾

You speak the words of choice, but be certain you really choose. Don't make decisions that are too fast for you but the right speed for someone else. Women talk of the men in their lives who want the cancer out and done with as fast as possible. In the pressure of the moment they comply; they see two doctors in two days, and within the week their breast is off. Spare yourself the anguish of pleasing others today and living with their decision for the rest of your life.

Cherish what is fundamental—your rights. It is necessary to take your time, to bring your mind and body together so that you are fully prepared. That is almost more important than what you choose.

Any choice is painful, but the most painful choice of all is living
with the one that someone else makes for us. I have
the right to choose my tomorrow.

Prophecy is the most gratuitous form of error.

—*George Eliot*

～

Like Disraeli, I now believe that there are "three kinds of lies: lies, damned lies, and statistics." Repeat this to yourself if you find yourself sinking under the inevitability of the odds. You are vulnerable and, worse than that, uninitiated in the world of numbers. Don't let the statistics come at you as hard realities. They aren't.

Statistics are an abstraction. As noted biologist Stephen Jay Gould (a cancer survivor who beat the odds) will tell you variation is nature's only true essence. So while statistics talk about averages and medians, they have no bearing on you as a "varying" individual.

Forget about the numbers. Why stifle your hope and will with numbers? All that counts is you and your attitude. You have a much bigger role to play than the passive calculation of average tendencies. All you have to do is be an individual.

As far as I am concerned, statistics have no bearing on me.

I will work in my own way, according to
the light that is in me.
—*Lydia Maria Child*

~

There is a divining power inside you. Focus inward. Notice fully and deeply your responses to all opinions. If two opinions differ, seek a third. If one in particular makes you angry, trust that reaction.

By holding both information and feeling inside you, without striving for a resolution, you best discover which opinion feels right. Once you have decided, don't be surprised if you find yourself angry at the doctor whose opinion you rejected. Emotionally, you are shouting, "How dare you upset me with the advice I have considered, but reject?" But this is exactly it, the decision-making process!

*Especially in the face of conflicting opinions, decision making
is a hard-won opportunity for me to grow.*

I'm not afraid of storms, for I'm learning
how to sail my ship.

—*Louisa May Alcott*

∼

The anxiety and self-questioning of a treatment choice may be agonizing at times, a feeling of being adrift at sea. It's not that you want to be told what to do, but there is the persistent, nagging feeling that you need more to go on, more coordinates, even when you know you have all the facts.

Accept that with the right to decide comes the responsibility of facing that there is no "right" answer.

*I push through the fear of making the wrong choice by sailing my
ship through the storm. There is no wrong choice if
I am steering the right course for myself.*

Flux

It was all happening in a great, swooping free fall,
irreversible, free of decision, in the full pull of gravity
toward whatever was to be.

—*Laura Z. Hobson*

~

The news and the rules kept changing from hour to hour
as different tests came in. I was sinking fast, unable to with-
stand the dramatic swings in my emotions. I wanted to
construct a decision, a plan, but my plans kept collapsing.

An elegant woman in the doctor's office told me she
was having her second mastectomy. She was undaunted,
elegant. I was very impressed.

How could she be so buoyant with a double mastectomy? I wasn't willing to accept just words. I wanted to see.
I asked her to show me, point-blank. She agreed.

I realize now that it wasn't what I saw—a reconstructed
breast—but that she was a reconstructed person. She told me
not to let cancer stop me. She herself had bought a new
business on the day she entered the hospital. I was elated.
I realized what I hadn't known moments before: If it had
to be a mastectomy, I could live with that, too.

*Today is wide open, as are my changing views about treatment
options; where there is flux, there is also the
possibility for new insights.*

35

Women like to sit down with trouble as if it were knitting.

—*Ellen Glasgow*

∾

If you feel caught in a cycle of indecision and fearfulness, try separating the overwhelming question before you into these two threads:

What is the significance of my breast to my experience of myself as a woman?

What are my attitudes toward cancer?

Now try to knit these two back together, interweaving your feelings about the cancer with the threat to your identity as a woman. What does the whole cloth say?

I rework my options today, dividing them into separate threads to craft into a decision.

A man must know how to defy opinion;
a woman how to submit to it.

—*Germaine de Staël*

～

The days of submitting are over! It is important for there to
be open and honest respect between doctor and patient.
But how do such ideal goals translate into the reality of a
working relationship, under pressure, time constraints, and
with the common perception of doctor as authority figure
and patient as someone who has to wait out in the waiting
room just like everyone else?

Say, "It is my life at stake and I am responsible for it."
When the time comes to ask questions about treatment options, perhaps even to question a point of authority or to express dissatisfaction with the level of attention you receive,
do it. This is all part of the back-and-forth flow of respect
and communication. This, too, is a part of your healing.

*I express my opinions to my doctor in a relationship
that fosters healing, communication, and respect.*

How forcible are right words.
—*The Holy Bible*

∾

In her book *In the Company of Others,* Jory Graham points out that when we are trying to sort out information, we tend to wring the full meaning out of every test and every word. Consciously or unconsciously, we have never been more attuned to the subtlety of language. The doctor says that in her opinion, "All things considered, your situation looks manageable," or "OK," "good," or "great." To the doctor, each of these words may describe the same basic result. But the positive or negative reinforcement in a doctor's offhand comment holds a lot of power.

I shall seek the kind of reinforcement I have a right to expect.

Interference

> It's queer how ready people always are with advice in any
> real or imaginary emergency, and no matter how many
> times experience has shown them to be wrong, they
> continue to set forth their opinions, as if they had
> received them from the Almighty!
>
> —*Annie Sullivan*

I was told by a woman who had refused all traditional treatment and instead opted to go down to Mexico to be healed
by touch that if I went ahead with my own plans I would
be nothing but cut, burned, and poisoned when it was all
over.

"Get out of my house," I screamed.

I was furious, but if you look at it closely, you'll see that
I agreed with her on one point at least: Belief in one's treatment, no matter what it is, is more than half the battle.

*I believe in the treatments I choose for myself. I can
only do for myself what works for me.*

It is the creative potential itself in human beings
that is in the image of God.

—*Mary Daly*

∼

I am a creative human being who will find imaginative
ways to deal with my fears as they come up. I summon my
creative energy in the direction of coping, rather than fear.
I am confident that I can live with the vagaries of the future. I now let go of resistance.

*By choosing to say yes to my treatment I am also choosing to let
go of my fear. Saying yes to my treatment is my best hope.*

Decision

The wave of the future is coming and there is no fighting it.
—Anne Morrow Lindbergh

∾

Your decision is frightening, but so is living with feelings of helplessness and uncertainty. Choosing relieves the anxiety of resisting going where you must go by bringing the mind and body together in a forward effort. Let a wave of peacefulness wash over you once you have successfully completed this task that was so hard to face. You have taken your step. Relax into the path you have chosen.

My decision is a relief. The peace I feel is born from my courage.

Surgery

Alone in the dark, I am going mad, counting my sorrows.
—*Chu Shu-chên*

∾

We are in the dark, except for knowing that our fear of the treatment has overtaken our fear of the disease.

It is very hard, when you feel well, to bring yourself to suffer. It is very hard, when you feel well, to choose to alter your body.

The process of choosing is a process of coming to terms with what you believe it is that you must do. Now is the time to let it be done.

When I see where I'm going, the obstacles don't get in my way.

It appears that even the different parts of the same person
do not converse among themselves, do not succeed
in learning from each other what are their
desires and their intentions.

—*Rebecca West*

∽

Surgery is a moment of truth. It brings together all the
questions and fears of the different parts of ourselves. If we
listen as we lie in our hospital bed, we hear a disjointed
monologue that Ionesco might have written, expressing
our conflicting fears.

*I fear cancer. I want it out. Surgery isn't hard—I'll be asleep.
How do I live with the surgery? Can anyone tell me now, before
they wheel me in, how it will change my life and my sense of myself as a woman? How can I worry about that when my life is at
stake? How can I live with a body that I might never again love?
Oh no, the gurney is coming. I'm scared.*

Acknowledge that the first stage in the resolution of your
personal crisis is surgery and that you have chosen it. Accept
that the surgery is a transitional phase and that you cannot
know its outcome. Face the challenge with courage. Forgive
yourself for your fears.

I welcome the surgery and shed tears for myself.

We one, must part in two. . . .
—*Christina Rossetti*

≈

The night before the surgery, I said goodbye to my breast all alone. I centered myself in the hospital bed and, with my hospital gown off, ran my hands up and down the sides of my body. It was a way to take in my body as it would be no more, intact and complete, with all its curves. My hands went around my breasts and in at the waist, out again at the hips and over my thighs.

I didn't worry about what was coming next or how I might feel the next day. I stayed right there in the moment. It was a peaceful and wistful farewell. Not angry or bitter, just sad. I was saying goodbye, letting go. It was a moving parting, like an embrace you see between two people who are forced to say goodbye under duress. I was both the soldier and his bride at wartime, tearfully bidding farewell.

I say goodbye to my breast, knowing that my farewell seeds a new beginning.

Shared Farewell

Noble deeds and hot baths are the best cures for depression.
—*Dodie Smith*

∽

My husband and I bathed together the night before. He soaped me down. And he addressed himself to my breast. "I loved your being here," he told it. Then we cried.

I trust that in looking back, even my goodbyes will be cherished.

Humor

❧

I used prayer and humor to get me through the surgery. My approach to prayer was personal, but for the humor I organized a contest among my friends. I asked them to give me their best jokes and I promised that the winning joke would be the one I told to the surgeon right before the operation.

Since both my doctor and I were golfers, I chose a golf joke. This is the last thing I said to him before I went under:

Four golfers were playing golf on Christmas Day. The first golfer said, "To get out to the course today, I had to give my wife a diamond ring." The second one countered, "I had to buy a trip to Hawaii." The third added, "I had to buy a new BMW." The fourth one looked confused. "I don't get it," he said. "I woke up this morning and just asked my wife which course she would prefer—golf or inter?" And she said, "Don't forget your sweater, dear."

In the operating room, don't forget to leave them laughing.

And what looks dark in the distance may brighten
as I draw near.

—*Mary Gardiner Brainard*

∽

This is it. Your hands are wrapped firmly inside the sheet, as if to tell you that you won't be needing them. Just let go, it is out of your control. Everything for the next several hours is up to the doctors and the nurses.

It is cold in there. You laugh to yourself that it's like a deep freeze and that we are, after all, meat. You recognize your doctor's warm and reassuring eyes behind the mask. You ask him to put you out before he puts the mask on, because the idea of the mask coming down on you feels frightening, a quirky legacy from childhood. You brace yourself gently. Say a prayer. Bid farewell to consciousness as you imagine a beautiful place that you visited once on vacation. You have done everything you can do.

My responsibility in the operating room is to make myself comfortable, laugh, pray, and finally, let go.

Anesthesia

Like water which can clearly mirror the sky and the trees
only so long as its surface is undisturbed, the mind can
only reflect the true image of the Self when it is
tranquil and wholly relaxed. . . .

—*Indra Devi*

~

Before going under, take yourself on an internal journey
to some favorite, serene place within you. Visualize it in
full detail, wherever you choose to go.

See azure seas and tropical fish running in schools just
beneath the water's surface. See white sand. Feel the warmth
of the sun. Notice the colors of the big striped towel that
you stretch yourself on. Run the time-worn pebbles through
your fingers as you listen to the gentle lapping of the waves.
Plan to stay in this peaceful place for the duration. It is
where you want to be while under anesthesia.

*I arrive into the anesthesia slowly. I get there on foot, on a peaceful
walk that ever so gradually descends into the white beach
and the blue sea of gentle sleep.*

You gave me wings to fly;
Then took away the sky.

—*Leonora Speyer*

∽

I fully expected that the surgery would be OK, that it would be an unmomentous event in my life. I was in my late 40s. I was married. I had nursed and raised my kids. But when I woke up in the hospital the day after the surgery with only one breast, I was devastated. I thought there would be no problem, but, oh, how I was wrong.

Who can ever accurately anticipate such feelings of loss? None of us. We must enter the hospital with the knowledge that we have begun a second emotional journey. We cannot predict what our emotions will be despite the certainty of our treatment choice or the nature of the treatment itself.

As they rise to the surface, I acknowledge my emotions on the morning after.

One reason our society has become such a mess is that
we're isolated from each other.

—Maggie Kuhn

We wake up to a hospital environment away from the
mainstream of our lives, far from the daily habits that define us. It is a place full of strangers, moving and acting according to a rhythm that is theirs, not ours. It is not unusual
to feel alienated or lonely, intimidated or frightened. Hospital
routines may infuriate us at times. Strange as they are, they
too will become familiar. Personalities will emerge from
among the staff, from among fellow patients; and our own
personalities will emerge.

I'll never forget the nurse who walked in, sat down on
the bed, and said, "So what's your story?" Or the one whom
I ended up comforting because she was afraid she might
have breast cancer herself.

The hospital is a community and while I'm there, I'm part of it.

Pain Medication

The world is wide, and I will not waste my life in friction
when it could be turned into momentum.

—*Frances Willard*

∿

A woman physician who has undergone mastectomy, radiation, and chemotherapy offers this advice: If you want
medication for pain, tell your doctor and the nurses to offer
you medication every three hours. That way if you lose
track of time, you will not run the risk of feeling pain before having your next dose. If you want to be more alert but
still guard against pain, ask your doctor to cut the dose but
maintain the frequency. Still other women prefer absolute
clarity, even when it includes discomfort.

*One woman's friction is another woman's momentum. I will be
clear about the level of medication I need and how it makes me feel.*

Control

When I'm in normal health, I'm a Presbyterian,
but just now I feel that even the wicked
get worse than they deserve.

—*Willa Cather*

~

The first person I wanted to talk to when I found myself flat
on my back in the hospital was the dietitian. I was appalled
by the stuff they were sending up to my room—white
bread, Jell-O. I insisted that someone come up and see me,
and together the dietitian and I worked out a diet that I
was willing to eat. They changed my diet immediately,
bringing me fish and whole-grain foods.

It was a victory. I had already made a commitment to a
diet that I trusted, and the last thing I wanted was to feel that
I was being sabotaged by the hospital. I demanded and got
control of my body despite being a patient in a large teach-
ing facility. Institutions are only impersonal if you allow
them to be. Breaking through that barrier of indifference
made all the difference to me.

It is striking how health-care institutions and the bodies
they repair seem to have diametrically opposed agendas.
To use Ms. Cather's word, you may feel you are being
treated wickedly. If you do, it is not wicked to in turn question the procedures to which you object. It is time to re-
assert your sense of dignity and question what you don't
like. It is time to take control.

I affirm my need for individuality and control.

Clothing

I'm a ragged individualist.
—*Jane Ace*

We all have many selves, and the one that seemed to emerge in the hospital was the rebellious kid in me. The whole time I was there, I insisted on wearing these silly, brightly colored striped anklet socks and a pair of ballet slippers, not to mention a once grand but now faded red satin robe in the boudoir tradition of old Hollywood movies.

I felt a need to express myself in whatever small ways I could, to assert my individuality, my identity. It seemed like a healthy notion, my desire to break out of the role of patient, which, despite my diagnosis, surgery, and five days in the hospital, felt very foreign.

At a time when I am trying to hold on to my essential self, clothing is as good a way as any to act out my individuality.

. . . It would be good to find some quiet inlet where the waters were still enough for reflection, where one might sense the joy of the moment, rather than plan breathlessly for a dozen mingled treats in the future.

—*Kathleen Norris*

∽

I only wanted to see a few friends and close family. I didn't want to get lost in a hubbub of activity. I didn't want distractions, because I felt it necessary to take time alone, to reflect and to focus. In a sense I was practicing a new way, the way in which I intended to live my life. That is how I saw my time in the hospital. I needed time to think. It was an opportunity to ask myself, what are the underlying meanings of this experience for my own life?

I reflect on the physical and emotional choices that will aid my recovery, and make them a part of my hospital stay.

. . . People seldom see the halting and painful steps by
which the most insignificant success is achieved.

—*Annie Sullivan*

∽

Surgery was like being hit by a Mack truck. Maybe it was
the morphine being fed to me intravenously, or maybe the
reconstructive device that I had inserted under my chest
wall at the time of my mastectomy.

As groggy as I was, I insisted on getting up. I don't know
why, but I felt my whole identity as a healthy woman rested
on flexing my muscles and using my body immediately.
Walking for me was purely a symbolic act. And the first
time I tried it, it was the hardest thing I ever did.

I set a goal of walking to the end of the hall and back. It
was maybe only 20 feet, but I was determined. And when
I got to the end of the hall and turned around, I thought I
heard the crowds cheering. As small a victory as it was on
the surface, it was a turning point for me.

I make exercise a goal, to speed my emotional as
well as physical recovery.

Drains

It is only in sorrow bad weather masters us, in joy
we face the storm and defy it.

—*Amelia Barr*

Mary woke up one rainy night in her hospital bed, very
wet. In a moment of terror, she thought her drain had
somehow ruptured. Groping in the dark, Mary assured herself that the drain was OK.

Still in the dark and flat on her back, even worse fears
flooded her mind. If it wasn't the drain, which would be bad
enough, she must be bleeding to death!

She quickly tried to reason, to calm herself. The mastectomy was on her left side, but it was her right arm that
felt so wet. There was no logical explanation.

She buzzed for the nurse but decided it was time to take
matters into her own hands. She got herself out of bed and
found the light. When she turned it on she started to laugh,
despite her initial terror. The hospital roof was leaking onto
her bed.

*Not only does life go on after breast cancer, but sometimes
it may literally intrude into my bed.*

God forgives those who invent what they need.
—*Lillian Hellman*

~

My way of dealing with the hospital stay was to think of myself as a tourist on vacation in a very strange hotel, one partial to fluorescent lights and people who look and feel lousy.

The hotel had a daily floor show and I was the star. I went on stage and got applause from my friends and family for having done so well. They brought flowers and celebrated me for being who I am. While I was in the hospital, the attention I received and the sheer effort of recovery kept me anchored and upbeat.

A hospital really is a way station, a place of transition that takes us out of our homes and hopefully surrounds us with equal doses of technology and tenderness. It prepares us for a return to life, because it is only when life normalizes that we start to fully experience the personal changes that have taken place.

Since I'm checked into this hotel, I might as well make the most of it.

... Use your imagination, try to visualize. ...
—*Charlotte Perkins Gilman*

I was in a panic, waiting for the pathology report and not knowing. So I decided to do something about it. I began mentally directing cancer cells out of my body on a regular basis, going through my system like some kind of haywire hausfrau with a vacuum cleaner combing through the wall-to-wall carpeting. Because without certain knowledge one way or the other, all you can be is afraid. Instead of letting myself be buffeted by wave upon wave of worry, I began to practice visualization. I combed through my body with my mind.

While I may bypass the need for further treatment, I cannot bypass the terror, dread, and fear of waiting for the pathology report.

Pathology Report

I am never afraid of what I know.
—*Anna Sewell*

After days of waiting, the doctor came in and told me what the pathology report said. There was lymph node involvement; I would need chemotherapy. I was frozen with fear.

I was overwhelmed, anticipating too much. So, I brought myself back to the present moment, to the pathology report. I let myself face my fear, face the facts of what I now knew in the moment. I would have chemotherapy. My fear was immediately supplanted by resolve and acceptance—not for cancer, but for what I knew I had to do next.

When you receive medical reports, remember that what you are feeling is not the pain of either disease or treatment. What you are feeling is fear.

How often do the clinging hands, though weak,
Clasp round strong hearts that otherwise would break.
    —*Mary Elizabeth Crouse*

∾

I get real mad when everyone comes into my room to visit and tells me, "Oh, you're a strong person. You're handling it." Well, hey! Can't I be weak once in a while, too?

I will be weak for today.

Leaving the Hospital

Dependency invites encroachment.
—*Patricia Meyer Spacks*

As much as we want to get out of the hospital, the prospect creates anxiousness and fear, too. It requires another leap, a resummoning of the energy to take back control over our lives, the very thing we were so reluctant to give up so recently. There are physical limitations and pain compounded by the responsibilities of home. While most of us have arranged for ways to cope—the help of friends, family, or professionals—there is still that small psychological threshold to reclaim and pass back through.

I look forward to leaving the hospital and facing the new challenges at home.

The delicate and infirm go for sympathy, not to the
well and buoyant, but to those who have
suffered like themselves.

—*Catharine Esther Beecher*

~

Once we are home from the hospital, the first emergency
is over—or so it may seem to the people around us. But for
us, the emergency has only deepened and is more fully felt.
Time and space open up into loneliness and feelings of
abandonment as sympathy and attentiveness drift away. In
the spaciousness of recovery, negative feelings may also
creep in: *Why hasn't he called? Where is everybody? Nobody
knows how I feel. How can I be so selfish and self-centered as to
feel forgotten by the very people who just rallied around me? Is it
fair to expect any more?*

Feeling forgotten or isolated is real. With everyone else
caught up in the bustle of work and play, it is easy to feel
left behind. Now is the time to look around. Look for the
many other women who share your immediate needs and
concerns so that you may offer each other the support you
need.

*I am now reaching out to other women through breast cancer
programs and support groups.*

Abandonment

My life will be sour grapes and ashes without you.
—Daisy Ashford

One never notices what has been done; one can only see
what remains to be done. . . .
—Marie Curie

When I was in the hospital, my friends were my main supports. When I got home, they still visited me, but back in the home environment they took to breast-feeding their children in front of me. It was as though once I was at home, the fact that I have lost a breast ceased being an issue. It felt like abandonment, that they could be so insensitive to me. The emergency may look like it's over to them, but I have yet to deal with my loss.

In the first weeks and months after surgery, I forgive my feelings of loss and abandonment at the same time that I forgive my friends.

Coping with Radiation and Chemotherapy

Faith

Faith is an excitement and an enthusiasm: it is a condition of
intellectual magnificence to which we must cling as to a
treasure, and not squander on our way through life in
the small coin of empty words, or in exact
and priggish argument. . . .

—*George Sand*

∿

With twelve positive lymph nodes, I need radiation and
chemotherapy. I want as much as I can get, because it is
my belief that it is my best way of living. I have a good
deal of trust in the treatment and in my physicians. I approach the treatment at the level of faith. Whatever they
suggest, I agree to do. I want to live, and I have faith that
this treatment is my ticket to a long life.

*To make a shadow disappear, sometimes you shine a
light on it, including the light of faith.*

Commitment

Everything is easy when we put our hearts into it.
—*Hroswitha of Gandersheim*

∾

If some say the process of receiving radiation treatment is easier than that of chemotherapy, there are also those who feel that radiation treatment is more of a commitment. It is a commitment of time in that you must show up five days a week for five or six weeks and that you live with it intimately. And it is a commitment in that the effects of radiation are permanent. Women often experience a tightening of the connective tissue on the chest wall, a permanent change to the body that does not fade away like the more transitory symptoms of fatigue. But first and foremost, radiation is a commitment to being well.

I accept that there is no "easy" treatment option and I choose that which will make me well.

Visualization

I am an explorer, then, and I am also a stalker,
or the instrument of the hunt itself.

—*Annie Dillard*

With radiation, I visualize little arrows going through my body and I see God as the hunter, pulling the bow, popping arrows into me to help me. I don't fear it.

I utilize visualizations to become an instrument of the hunt.

Anger

Why am I idiotically timid before such people, while
at the same time so critical of their limitations?

—Nadine Gordimer

≈

I didn't feel that I was getting the attention I deserved, as
though the technician I saw daily thought that lumpectomy and radiation were no big deal. It made me angry.

I know that lumpectomy with radiation is a less obviously disfiguring treatment, but there are still all the
underlying questions: How did this happen to me? Did
they get it all? And the truth is that I still feel a terrible
sense of loss.

The next day, I spoke up. The technician blushed deep
red. She had no idea how I was feeling. The emotions were
so high, there were tears in our eyes. She told me I had
just made her a better health professional. And I told her she
just made me a stronger person.

*The degree of physical change to my body is not a barometer of my
emotional reaction. When I feel I am not getting the sensitivity
I deserve, I have a right to express my anger about this.*

Then give to the world the best you have,
And the best will come back to you.

—Madeline Bridges

∼

Radiation treatments are a daily reminder of cancer. I felt I couldn't get away from cancer, when every day radiation summoned me backwards instead of on with life. But gradually, day by day, I started to open up. I started to see another side. I began to recognize the faces and the stories of the other women who received regular treatments alongside me. I got to know the doctors and the nurses and staff. I focused on these relationships and how they grew over the days and weeks. I came to see my treatments as a daily shared effort toward wellness.

When I open up to the supportive relationships all around me, I welcome my daily treatments.

Active Patient

> The beauty of the world has two edges, one of laughter,
> one of anguish, cutting the heart asunder.
>
> —*Virginia Woolf*

∾

I was between Radiation and Oncology, waiting to have a blood workup, so I decided to stay in a hospital gown. Boldly, like an active patient, I took the elevator upstairs, holding my blouse, bra, and prosthesis. It did take courage to decide something so small, because you can't help feeling vulnerable in a skimpy hospital gown when you've had a mastectomy.

While I was waiting upstairs, a nurse came up to me and asked if I wore a prosthesis. I thought she wanted to see it, so I said yes. Then she handed me my prosthesis and said, "Here, you dropped this in the lobby." Still, I congratulated myself for being an active patient, seeking ways to ease my own treatment and discomfort.

*When I am an active patient, it is OK when some of the
minor details occasionally slip through my fingers.*

... Necessity also is an object of exploration.
—*Simone Weil*

∾

The first cycle of chemotherapy treatment is the hardest, going through it as we are by necessity and not knowing what to expect. Desperate questions such as *What is it like?* and *What can I do about the side effects?* remain unanswered until the first direct experience.

With the first treatment behind us, however, it is already time to experiment. A good place to start is with the best time of day for treatment. Some women have discovered that by taking the drugs at night—and by bunching them up—they feel much better the next afternoon and evening. Also experiment with the sequence of anti-anxiety and anti-nausea drugs taken before chemo. If you feel too jumpy from some of the medication, try taking the relaxant last. Experiment with different nausea drugs until you discover the best for you.

As an active patient, I explore ways to meet the treatment commitment I have made.

There is nothing colder than chemistry.
—*Anita Loos*

Self-programming and self-talk are treatment supports. Before treatment, even in the car on the way there, talk to yourself in simple and direct terms. "I can do this. This will make me well." The best way to prepare for treatment is to overcome fear and negative associations by positively shaping your perceptions about what you are about to undertake: "This is a medicine that makes me well. When I receive chemotherapy it will be as a golden elixir going after my cancer cells."

To relax myself during treatment, I begin by relaxing myself before treatment.

Woes have their ebb as well as flood.
—*Katherine Fowler Philips*

Each time I physically show up at the doctors', all the feelings about having breast cancer resurface. It is the realization, once again, that I have a serious disease. So each time, I go through the mourning process. It's the time in the cycle when I worry and get scared. But that's OK. It's important to let these scared feelings come. What I feel now can't hurt me later, so I welcome the ritual purge.

I am aware that the amount of control I have,
like everything in life, ebbs and flows.

I endeavor . . . to be wise when I cannot be merry, easy
when I cannot be glad, content with what cannot be
mended and patient when there is no redress.

—*Elizabeth Montagu*

∾

After the needle has gone in, ask for a blanket. Bundle up
and begin:

Start with your toes. Focus on them and relax them.
Then your feet, ankles, calves, thighs, all the way up to
your head. When your body is relaxed, take it on a relaxation journey.

Visualize a big black sky and way out there in the distance
a yellow blinking light. Focus on the light, and as it gets
nearer, see that it says RELAX. Watch as the words gently
pulse, dimming and brightening. Watch the pulsing yellow light transmute into a golden sun above a white sand
beach. See yourself stretched out there. Let the sand con-
tour to your body. Listen to the waves and let the sun warm
you with the whitest part of its light. Feel how that warmth
becomes one with and accompanies the golden elixir of
the treatment. Imagine how the sunlight and the elixir together are coursing through your body, eliminating cancer cells and warming you into a state of relaxed and satisfied
sleep.

I am so warmed by this relaxation, I fall asleep during treatment.

She always says, my lord, that facts are like cows. If you look them in the face hard enough they generally run away.

—*Dorothy L. Sayers*

❧

The week before a chemotherapy treatment, I always have some new imaginary symptom of metastatic disease because anticipating the treatment sets me up to think about cancer more. When feeling vulnerable, the imagination has an amazing capacity to cook up terrible thoughts about the state of my health. So I tell myself over and over that these are not facts, but fears.

Fear can make cows and pains look a lot bigger and more threatening than they need to be.

Clouds behind clouds in long succession rise. . . .
—*Anna Letitia Barbauld*

There is an organic depression that accompanies chemotherapy, one that goes well beyond the fact that you might already have good reason to be depressed. It is not the sort of depression that you can will yourself out of, but three or four days later it passes like a cloud. The solace is knowing in advance that during this period you are much more prone to fear and to negative thoughts until suddenly you feel alive again.

It is physical, so much so that some days you don't want to get up, as though depression has gotten into your bones. All you can do is tell yourself that you are "in the chemo" and be tolerant. Wait and notice when it lifts. It is easy to blame yourself for your feelings—but don't. Blame the drugs! The cloud of depression that follows treatment is physiological and chemical. It is not strictly emotional.

On the days when I am "in the chemo," I will look
forward to the days when I am out of it.

Scalp Treatment

I have heard say the executioner is very good,
and I have a little neck.

—*Anne Boleyn*

It gets so I wish I could just get my head chopped off. My scalp and hair are so dried by the drugs that my head really hurts. It's not pain exactly, but soreness. Over-the-counter oil treatments for dry hair help and can continue even after all hair is lost. Sleeping on a satin pillow is another secret. These are small things, but it's the sort of things that the doctors don't mention and that can make a big difference.

Before I consider chopping my head off, I'll talk with other women and find out how they cope.

I can remember walking as a child. It was not customary
to say you were fatigued. It was customary to
complete the goal of the expedition.

—*Katharine Hepburn*

Despite the chemotherapy, I incorporate exercise into my
routine. The exercise helps me sleep, helps me combat the
depression from the chemotherapy and the depression from
what I'm going through. Exercise stimulates blood flow
and delivers the chemotherapy to all points in my body. It
makes the chemo more effective. I see exercise as a way to
fight the cancer. Sometimes it's hard, but afterwards I feel
vibrant and alive. It's a healthy kind of tired, not the tired
of chemotherapy. And at the same time, it keeps the rest of
my body looking good. Moving my body, enabling the
chemo, and meeting my personal goal are all good for my
self-esteem.

*I look forward to the physical and emotional challenges of
today and have the strength to meet them because I exercise.*

Prayer

Loving, like prayer, is a power as well as a process.
It's curative. It is creative.

—*Zona Gale*

I let the doctors do their work and I pray to be helped through this experience. And I have everyone I know pray for me. I don't care who or what they are. I have a Catholic prayer chain that my sister organized in the East; I have a Methodist family praying for me in the Midwest and a Buddhist bell-ringing ceremony through a friend in California. If whistling "Dixie" would work, I would use it all. I urge every woman to take advantage of spirituality. Each of us needs to be supported and uplifted by exploring prayer and finding our own way into the spiritual realm.

All forms of prayer join together in a single wave of peacefulness.
I step into that wave and let it wash over me.

Leaving aside the bough that produced beauty's fruit,
Inclining toward a bough that no such fruit does show.

— *Wallada*

As premenopausal women facing chemotherapy, what crashes in on us is the temporary, if not the certain, loss of fertility. This is a loss that has nothing to do with whether we ever planned to bear children, or whether we have already borne all that we wished. It is still a cut to the fabric in which we, as women, cloak ourselves.

Feminine identity is woven from many things, including fertility and the possibility of bearing fruit like boughs of a tree. Yet femaleness transcends fertility and breasts; it is an essence that cannot be lost.

Today I mourn my losses at the same time that I celebrate that I am a woman with courage and tears to cry.

Necessity can set me helpless on my back, but she cannot keep me there; nor can four walls limit my vision.

—*Margaret Fairless Barber*

I don't sit around and store up energy. If I have it, I use it and then I rest. I go all out. Then I sleep. I'd rather do what I can now. I suppose it's the principle of living in the present moment. Whatever I have, I use. I use it now.

Expending the energy I have may be counted as a victory.

Humor

The worst in life, we are told, is compatible with the
best in art. So too the worst in life is compatible
with the best in humour.

—*Agnes Repplier*

On a good day between chemotherapy treatments, I went
with friends to look over the ocean from the cliffs. Need I
say more? My wig blew off and tumbled down and my
friends went after it. All I remember is snippets of conversation wafting up on the wind: "Is that it? No, that's not it.
What's that? Oh my god, that's a cat!" All I can say is that
you have to have a sense of humor in order to be well.

*When I bring a sense of humor to the worst situations
in my life, even I can't help but laugh.*

They were mortal, but they were unconquerable.
—*Willa Cather*

~

When I began chemo, I marked all the dates that I was to receive treatment on a calendar. Midway through, I got a call telling me my date would have to be rescheduled because my doctor had left the clinic. What they were telling me was that some new doctor whom I had never met was going to inject these chemicals into me, and on a day that was convenient for him and inconvenient for me!

I flew into a rage. I wrote a letter to the head of the center telling him that he had damn well better get that new doctor off the golf course so I could meet him before my next treatment, and that as far as I was concerned that treatment was going to take place on nothing but the appointed date, which of course it did.

Anger turned to action works very well in my
gaining control over treatment.

Coping with Blood Counts

Fiction reveals truths that reality obscures.

—*Jessamyn West*

~

The double effect of radiation and chemotherapy treatments—the "echo" effect—can bring blood counts way down. The doctor told me that my blood count was down to "one" and I ended up in the hospital. His words alarmed me because it made me think of having only one white blood cell in my whole body. I turned that "one" around into one huge, powerful cell as big as my whole body, and that is what I fought with.

> *A positive attitude toward setbacks in my treatment comes down to one—and that one is me.*

Though we be sick and tired and faint and worn,
Lo, all things can be borne!

—*Elizabeth Chase Akers*

∾

There may be a cumulative effect with nausea and fatigue. Concentrate on the fact that this, too, is time limited. As the fatigue level rises, it is time to reduce expectations of yourself. Comparison to pre-chemo days is irrelevant. Instead, see everything you do as a victory. Be pleased with yourself and, most of all, be forgiving of yourself.

I rejoice in whatever I have done today.

I have found that sitting in a place where you have
never sat before can be inspiring.

—*Dodie Smith*

I am sharing my chemotherapy experiences with other
women who are doing the same. One of us has just had a
recurrence. Fear of recurrence is not the problem; the need
to make sense of it is. It has forced all of us to think about
recurrence in ourselves and to imagine what it would be
like. It is very frightening to try on a worst-case scenario,
but I have had to explore it. And what happens is that you
say, "No! That's not what I want for myself." By letting
yourself descend into the fear, you come up out of it
strengthened, motivated, and inspired.

*When I descend into fears of recurrence, I emerge
strengthened and motivated.*

In violent and chaotic times such as these, our only chance
for survival lies in creating our own little islands of sanity
and order, in making little havens of our homes.

—*Sue Kaufman*

∾

My favorite thing to do is to sit around and read books.
And although chemotherapy is tough, it also gives me permission. I am the mother of two sons. My boys tell me to
get up and do something. Maybe that works for them and
for my husband, that masculine need to 'do,' but it doesn't
work for me. I hold firm with my own way of coping,
which is to be still and calm and to read books. I don't have
to do anything.

*Trusting my intuition about how much I want to do is
the way to get through the treatment process.*

Travel not only stirs the blood . . . It also gives
strength to the spirit.

—*Florence Prag Kahn*

⁓

Travel is a healing distraction. It slows down time to a pace
we recollect from youth, when everything in the world is
new and the days are full and long, filled with the excitement of first discovery. It heals us with distraction in the
same way that a call from a boyfriend seemed to cure us of
a headache years and years ago. Travel is a journey into
and away from the self. So enjoy yourself, but be prepared
for all eventualities, even a wig for that morning when your
head might come up off the hotel pillow while your hair
stays put.

I welcome travel as a way of going outside myself.

If one sticks too rigidly to one's principles one
would hardly see anybody.

—*Agatha Christie*

∼

I am a very social person. People are my sustenance. But
going through chemotherapy, I planned for life to stop.
That doesn't work. I think the key is to have your life re-
semble what it was before as much as possible. It's not denial, it's life as usual, but with allowances made.

For instance, every year we have a big Christmas party
and this year was no different. Only I renamed it. It wasn't
a Christmas party, but a cancer party. That is, it was an affirmation of life party, and I had a wonderful time.

Whenever I feel up to it, I will enjoy people and celebrate life.

Goals

This shall be my parting word—know what you want to
do—then do it. Make straight for your goal and go
undefeated in spirit to the end.

—Ernestine Schumann-Heink

I have room in my life for chemotherapy treatment and
one other major activity. I have made it my child, not my
work. Or perhaps a better way to say it is that my child is
my work. My child is my way of structuring time, forgetting cancer treatment, maintaining normalcy, and foster-
ing a sense of accomplishment.

*I am taking care of two things today and at least one
of them is myself.*

In some situations, to be polite—is enough.

—*Gisela Richter*

～

I hate it when peole ask, "How are you feeling?" You know they mean well, but once you have had cancer and are undergoing treatment those words become charged. I feel as if I'm being checked up on, as though the asker is ghoulishly expectant of bad news or, worse still, as though he or she knows something that I don't.

It is an eerie feeling being asked how you feel. It makes me feel like I am this disease. The irony is that I have always felt well. It is only the treatments that have made me feel poorly.

The next time someone asks me, "How are you feeling?"
I will feel all these feelings and say, "Why, I'm fine,
thank you. How are you?"

Motherhood and Chemotherapy

What a difference it makes to come home to a child.
—Margaret Fuller

∾

Having a one-year-old helps me along. She's learning about life and excited about everything. She reminds me how wonderful life can be. There's so much to do with her that it normalizes my life as I go through the treatment. She doesn't give me any slack; she hasn't a clue about cancer.

Of course it's tiring. I have to surrender her for big chunks of time after each treatment when all I can do is rest and observe her. But it's its own reward. At the end of the day I don't know if I'm tired from the cancer treatment or if I'm tired from being the mother of a one-year-old, and I think to myself, *Isn't that wonderful?*

Every day that I get to be a mother is a bonus day, a day of fulfillment and the reward of being a parent.

Sure of nothing but our dying . . .
—*Veronica Gambara*

∼

There are times during chemotherapy, like around three in the morning, when you have to push and fight and talk to yourself.

Make tapes. Use your voice to record visualizations that help you through the middle of the night. Try the theme "I want to see the year 2000." Listen to it over and over again and it will get you through. Talking to yourself is the light that brings on the dawn.

And if there's someone there beside you, I say hug and cry together until you've had enough of crying. Trust that your fears can be tamed by daylight, because when the light comes they are gone, you are sorry about the red eyes, and you decide that life and laughter are a lot more fun.

*I am now talking myself from depression to fortitude,
from darkness to light and into the year 2000.*

"But then what did you want me to forgive you for?"

"I wanted you to forgive me for being mean," he said, "and having to be what I am, and do what I have done." A smile passed over his lips. "Just as you might ask me to forgive you for being you."

—*Rebecca West*

We may think that we need to ask forgiveness for being ourselves at times, on those days when we feel like we could jump out of our skin except that we're too tired. We snap. We are irritable and restless.

Some women are frustrated that their usual remedies don't work at such times. They figure they'll play it safe and relate to something easy and passive, like reading a book. But restlessness and irritability resurface. Maybe watching a short television show is about the closest thing to fit our mood, something that moves and changes quickly, that mirrors our own restlessness.

So tune in and zone out. Maybe there is no better way to get through these periods than as a restless couch potato. It's OK. It's what happens. And it's OK to ask your doctor for something to alleviate the symptoms.

I forgive myself for being the restless and irritable self that the drugs sometimes cause me to be.

... What has become of your eyes, your ears,
your memories?

—*George Sand*

A very close friend called to say that she was going to visit
me from quite a long distance away. I know the very idea
of it would have given me great pleasure. But when she
showed up at my door, I had absolutely no recollection of
any such conversation. I was surprised to see her. That sort
of memory loss seems to happen a day after the chemo.
But the loss is temporary and occurs only at the time you
are the least well.

I will remember that it is OK to forget.

A time comes when one is forced to concentrate on living.
—*Colette*

∼

I went to work during chemotherapy. My head wasn't always there, but my body was. It was important for me to have to show up and present a good face, even if my business partner had to check all my figures a second time.

> *Even if chemotherapy leaves me foggy, I hold onto the clarity of what I plan to accomplish.*

Triumph

The distant strains of triumph
Burst agonized and clear!
—*Emily Dickinson*

~

On the day I took my last pill, I ceremoniously carried the vial outside into the backyard and smashed the hell out of it with a hammer. It was very cleansing, a clear delineation of the end of a hellish period in my life. It is good to do that sort of thing, to acknowledge the rage and grief with impromptu ceremonies of triumph and completion.

I celebrate my willingness to express my feelings at the end of chemotherapy and the creativity with which I act them out.

> . . . Concern should drive us into action,
> not into a depression.
>
> —*Karen Horney*

~

We celebrate the end of treatment. But another tiny voice, one we can hardly believe we hear, talks to us in fearful moments. "I am left on my own," it says. "I don't see the doctor again for months. If I am happy, why am I anxious and scared?"

There is a sense of connectedness and hope in the process of receiving treatment, unpleasant as the treatments may be. Conversely, there is loss in its completion. We are cut off from our doctor, momentarily frightened, and alone again in the face of the unknown.

Face these feelings and act in whatever way necessary. A beginning might be to soften the transition by reaching out for support from your doctor or nurse by phone.

Today I think creatively about how to answer the little voices of fear and depression that accompany the end of treatment.

If things happen all the time you are never nervous; it is
when they are not happening that you are nervous.

—*Gertrude Stein*

∾

I hate checkups. I am always terrified. I feel like I live on
a little umbilical cord attached to my oncologist and that I'm
allowed three-month reins. My solution is to always go in
there with the same cocky attitude. I think to myself, "If
you're trying to find something wrong, doc, I won't let
you. I am a very healthy person who just happens to have
had this disease. So if you don't mind my saying so, damn
you, doc."

*The process of having gone through cancer and survived has its joys
. . . and checkups. Having handled the cancer, I know
I can handle the checkups.*

....

Body and Self

Fighting back. On a multiplicity of levels, that is
the activity we must engage in. . . .
—*Susan Brownmiller*

It wasn't until I had a mastectomy, when everybody who was touching me was a stranger again, putting stuff on my arms, leaning on me, that I made the connection: it was like the experience of rape. I got in there and I started shaking like I've never shook in my life, and crying uncontrollably—raw feeling like I've never had. I have had both experiences and I can say that mastectomy brings up similar reactions, that sense of having one's body invaded by strangers.

*Mastectomy is an invasion of my body and my self-esteem,
leaving visible and invisible wounds that need to heal.*

O Friend, I fear the lightest heart makes sometimes
heaviest mourning.

—*Caroline Sheridan Norton*

I took a walk through a meadow that goes down to some cliffs. As I walked, I felt many layers come off me, mother, workaday person, wife, all of them gone. Then the tears came. What I felt was true regret for my body and what happened to it. It was not going to be pretty anymore. I faced that fact. I mourned mentally for that aspect of the breast cancer experience, all by itself. I was sorry, really sorry about what had happened to me and what I had lost.

Today I take a walk alone and strip away the layers
until I get down to mourning.

The inevitability of gradualness . . .
—*Beatrice Potter Webb*

≈

We mourn the loss of a breast as we mourn the death of any loved one. And while that process is ongoing, we begin to mourn not only what is gone, but also what is left behind.

Coming to terms with what is left—our new selves—is also a process. Little tests like standing before a mirror, trying on new or old clothing, exposing ourselves to friends, to lovers, to strangers, and talking about ourselves and cancer, are all part of the process of rebuilding self-image and self-esteem through contact with life. It is how we rediscover that despite all that has happened, our truest selves persist.

What is most important about the process of rebuilding my self-image and self-esteem is that I begin it.

Confrontation

∼

I was looking for a way to confront the issue of my body image head on. I vowed to myself that I would enroll in a massage class, knowing full well that part of the time the students are nude and that I would be exposing myself, with only one breast, to all these strangers. I was looking for a nonsexual forum in which to confront both men and women. I wanted to be completely accepted the way I was. I knew that whether or not I opted for reconstruction, first I wanted to be sure that it wasn't just to fit into somebody's mold of how I should look. In the end, it was a painful test for me, something that I would suggest others do a bit more gradually.

*I recognize that not every test of my body image
need be an outright confrontation.*

... the inner spirit, the inner voice; the human compulsion
when deeply distressed to seek healing counsel within
ourselves, and the capacity within ourselves both to
create this counsel and to receive it.

—*Alice Walker*

I set up a program. Every day I spent about 15 minutes
looking in the mirror. It was one aspect of rebuilding my
body image. It was like getting to know a new friend. I
approached myself openly, honestly, and with love. I made
daily visual and physical contact with myself through the reflection in the mirror. Sometimes I just looked. Sometimes
I talked out loud to myself. Sometimes I rubbed cream
onto my scar, or touched the area around it. Sometimes I
tried on clothes to see how they looked, what worked and
what didn't. Gradually I came to know, recognize, accept,
and even love myself once again. It did not happen
overnight. But then, what long-lasting relationship does?

*I look in the mirror and study myself every day and say, "That
is just me there. I am no better or worse. It is just me."*

. . . The burden is so heavy just now, the task is so great,
that reinforcement is needed.
—*Mary McLeod Bethune*

I have been forced to acknowledge the impact of chemotherapy, radiation, and surgery to my body and my spirit. It is not any single one of them, but all of them together that has been so physically and emotionally devastating. In an odd way, it is like that period of time after just having a baby—total exhaustion and the hardest time to get back on one's feet comes exactly when the most demands on us are being made. It's a double or triple whammy. I'm so tired and yet there's so much to do, so much work that needs to take place on my physical and emotional self. Yes, it's just like having a baby, except that the baby who needs the caring and the mother who does the nursing are all rolled into one.

This is a caring and loving process in which I give myself
permission to take the time and the rest I need.

When one is stranger to oneself then one is
estranged from others too.

—*Anne Morrow Lindbergh*

It is natural to have feelings of fear and of self-rejection as
we get to know our altered bodies and altered selves once
again. What is important is to not defend too long against
those feelings, because at some point, to avoid is a form of
denial.

To really look at ourselves, inside and out, is a courageous act. Difficult as it is for some women, it is always the
beginning point, the first step in the process of self-healing.

*My fear of looking at myself is just one more measure of my
courage. I accept that I can look and be afraid
all at the same time.*

. . . Our concern must be to live while we're alive—
to release our inner selves from the spiritual death that
comes with living behind a facade designed to conform
to external definitions of who and what we are.

—Elisabeth Kübler-Ross

I drove up to the Outer Banks of North Carolina. I checked
into a motel room and would not come out. I was afraid to
do anything, afraid to even walk on the beach. I was that
insecure, that needful of hiding, of covering up my exis-
tence. I actually worried that someone might rape me! It
wasn't the rape itself I feared, but my fantasy that the rapists
would stop in the middle of the act when they saw how
strange I looked under my clothes.

After two days, I asked myself, *Why am I afraid to leave this
room? Why am I afraid to walk on the beach?* I had to sit and
talk to myself and reassure myself about what I was capable of doing. In calling up that other voice, I finally summoned my strength and walked out. Oddly enough,
stepping over that threshold was my first step in rebuilding
my self-esteem.

*However I define my own first step, I am capable
of crossing that threshold.*

There are no accusers; there could be no judge.
—*Selma Lagerlöf*

∽

I lived with a roommate named Judy for two years and she never knew I had had a mastectomy. I have been on business trips with women and have shared a room with them for days and they never knew. The most important thing for me is to keep it a secret—a big, dark, dank secret. It's not the issue of breasts, but of being different. I feel freakish. I don't tell other women because I'm afraid I'll feel judged. But I know it's really me who is the judge and who has yet to accept her own body.

Today I challenge the cycle of silence and denial that is the barrier to my feelings of self-worth.

Adolescence is just one big walking pimple.
—*Carol Burnett*

~

With mastectomy and chemotherapy it is as though we have become teenagers again, preoccupied with and uncertain about our appearance. Just as when we were girls, we find ourselves face to face with major body changes. Instead of the development of breasts, body hair, and menstruation, we face the opposite: loss or reduction of one or both of our breasts, possible loss of hair, and the early onset of menopause.

Our breasts, our hair, and our periods are valued and sexually charged parts of ourselves. They are old friends that have come to define our sense of feminine integrity. Then suddenly they are gone! Cancer is invisible to us, but the changes to our bodies are not. And like teenagers once again, we question our worth, who we are, and why anyone should find us either valuable or attractive.

Given all that I have been through, it is no wonder that I feel as uncertain and insecure as a teenager.

. . . Perhaps we have not fully understood that anger
is a secondary cover for hurt.

—*Charlotte Painter*

Jane expressed a deepening joy for all that she had experienced since her diagnosis and treatment, even the difficult and the sad, and the struggles with herself and her body. But in the middle of reflecting on what she had learned about herself, her face turned red and she kicked a chair with all her might. "Some days, I'd give all my insight back in a second. It makes me damn angry, because with all I've come to learn and understand, life may still go on without me!"

*I see my illness as an opportunity rather than a tragedy,
but some days I am just plain angry.*

> . . . True emancipation begins neither at the polls
> nor in courts. It begins in woman's soul.
>
> —*Emma Goldman*

~

Visualize that you are a little girl of about six or seven. Look at her. See all the good things in her, her sparkling eyes and creativity, her openness, her needs. If she is crying, comfort her. Now make her very, very small and take her and put her in your heart.

Every time your feelings about yourself hurt, make yourself that tiny girl again, and put her in your heart. If she is crying, comfort her. Then encase her there.

When you are being hard on yourself, place yourself back in your heart and give yourself the love you need. If you imagine others are judging you, look at them and encase them in your heart as well.

*Self-love is self-healing. I provide it for myself. I have
something to offer and it is love.*

> I beheld the wretch—the miserable monster I had created.
> —*Mary Wollstonecraft Shelley*

I was on a crosstown bus on the way to see my doctor and this woman got on. Even though it was the middle of the day, she was decked out in an unbelievable dress that could only be described as stretch gold lamé. It doesn't matter that she looked ridiculous, the point is that she was falling out of the dress. I could see that she was eccentric, strange. But that didn't matter. I wanted what she had: two healthy breasts! I hated her. I thought she was a monster for walking around like that, even if she was a monster that I created.

> *I stay with what I feel. Sometimes it may be*
> *"Why me and why not her?"*

She always believed in the old adage: "Leave them
while you're looking good."

—Anita Loos

~

I have gotten very cocky now that my hair is back. I've
been wearing a hat, which makes me feel more complete,
more finished. And it gives me attitude. I flirted with a
man just last week—just a few words, a few glances. It was
liberating to realize that he didn't know anything about me
or cancer and that I didn't have to explain it to him or to
anybody else. For those few minutes it was behind me. I am
starting to see myself in a new way, looking forward to
even more contact with the world.

*I experience how my self-image and self-esteem continually
alter and change, and with them, my view of the world.*

The motto should not be: Forgive one another; rather,
Understand one another.

—Emma Goldman

I got myself a sign that says *Shit Happens* and I hung it up at home where I could see it every day. I'm not the type that walks around in sweatshirts proclaiming my thoughts, or who covers my car with bumper stickers, but that saying, vulgar as it is, has come to hold real significance for me. It means that I didn't get cancer because I was a bad person.

For a long time I felt like I was being punished, that developing breast cancer was my fault. I don't buy those thoughts anymore. I have met so many lovely women, talented and successful women, women of all descriptions, who have had breast cancer. Nobody can convince me that they have all brought this down on themselves. Knowing them has been a validating experience for me. The sad fact is that shit happens.

*Today I pick a phrase to live by, write it down, and hang it up
where I can look at it and validate myself every day.*

. . . The more revolutions occur, the less things change.
                                    —*Georgie Anne Geyer*

The way I have preserved my sense of identity is to spend
my time talking about what I always spent my time talking
about, things other than cancer. I am about art and litera-
ture and politics and newest loves, not cancer. That's who
I am on the inside and that's who and what I continue to
be.

I liked myself before breast cancer and I continue to like myself now.

People need joy quite as much as clothing.
Some of them need it far more.

—*Margaret Collier Graham*

Following mastectomy, I purchased one plain, cheap prosthesis bra. I only bought one because I thought I wouldn't live long enough to need another.

At a support group, I noticed a bit of lace on someone's bra. When she said she had a prosthesis in it, I asked if I could see the bra, and I was absolutely stunned at how pretty it was.

This little encounter proved to me that it's not so much what happens but how each of us treats what happens that is so critical in how we feel about ourselves. That lady had been through exactly what I had, but she dressed herself with joy.

*I am good enough to enjoy a pretty bra, even if it does
have only one breast in it.*

The pain of the discipline is short, but the glory
of the fruition is eternal.
—*Harriet Beecher Stowe*

∼

I use ballet as a form of exercise, a discipline, and a way of
getting control back over my body and my life. The music
is beautiful. It makes me feel graceful, and I've learned to
stand proud and to stand tall. By taking ballet, or any form
of exercise, a woman regains a sense of balance. I mean
that in the physical sense but more importantly, in the emotional sense.

Exercise is a way of gaining control over my body and my life.

Love is a great beautifier.
—*Louisa May Alcott*

When I became bald I was like Samson. Somehow my self-worth and my emotional strength seemed to all be rooted in my scalp. I grieved in the way you might grieve over the loss of someone you love. My husband took me by the shoulders and said, "Look at me. I'm the man that you love and I am bald."

He was right. So what if I'm bald? So is he. And my hair is going to grow back, which is more than he can say. Yet, I love him anyway. He is wonderful in my eyes, and knowing that, I finally realized that I still had some value too.

Today I make a list of all the people I love without hair
and put my own name at the top.

Feedback

Tricia said that she liked the way I looked better than the way she looked. That shocked me entirely. Up until that point I thought of myself as an amputee or deformed or chopped off, all images of having been drastically altered. Tricia is one of those women who always imagines herself as a movie star, all streamlined and upright and none of the saggy stuff that is the reality of women's breasts. Leave it to Tricia, who has two healthy breasts, to find my fake versions preferable to the real thing. But I couldn't thank her enough. I came away from our little session of show and tell believing I wasn't amputated or cut off. Suddenly I was upright, firm, and forever young from my neck to my navel. Her words, her perspective, gave me a new way of looking at myself.

I borrow the words and perspectives of others to help re-form my self-image and feelings of self-esteem.

I know I'm not exactly a bombshell, but one has to
make the best of what one's got.

—*Joan Sutherland*

My solution to being knocked off kilter in terms of my
self-image and self-esteem was to develop one of my really violent crushes—on my doctor! I know it sounds adolescent, but I take the feeling seriously. What could be more
affirming? OK, so he's my doctor. But he is the only man
who has seen me naked besides my husband, and why
shouldn't I have a crush on him? He's told me all the things
I need to hear: that I'm courageous, that I have a forceful
life spirit, and that I'm not fat and not ugly and not worth-
less. On all those levels it seems a very healthy thing. I feel
a sense of pride that I have managed to come up with this
neat little creative solution right in the midst of my crisis.

My infatuations may be the beginnings of my acceptance of self.

Intention

The biggest sin is sitting on your ass.
—*Florynce R. Kennedy*

∿

Intention is a powerful tool. It is how we articulate and create what we want. If we *intend* to improve our feelings of self-worth and self-esteem, we are taking responsibility. Regardless of the specific decisions and actions we take for ourselves, taking responsibility goes a long way. It is our antidote to feelings of anger at ourselves and at the world.

Intention may come in the form of reconstruction, of exposing ourselves to our friends, of joining a support group, of tattooing over our mastectomy scar and mailing a photograph of it to all of our friends. From the cautious to the outrageous, the underlying message is that we are intending to grab our insecurities by the horns and wrestle them to the ground as dramatically or deliberately as we can.

My intention is to test myself by moving myself out of my safe zone in whatever way I can.

Affirmation

I know we grow more lovely
Growing wise.
—*Alice Corbin*

Cancer is emotionally and physically shattering, but it is also an opportunity to see. By breaking me open, it has shown me that my body is just my body and that I am what's inside. What I love is what's inside. And what others love about me is what's inside as well.

Today, I look at the inner and outer me with the clarity that cancer affords.

Reconstruction

... One never discusses anything with anybody who can
understand, one discusses things with people
who cannot understand. ...

—*Gertrude Stein*

Many women report that their partners discourage them
from elective reconstructive surgery out of a kind of loving protectiveness. Those feelings are to be appreciated,
but we must recognize that it is hard for anyone else to
measure the psychological necessity of such an operation
for us. We are the only ones who know our own internal
pressure to restore feelings of wholeness in terms of breast
symmetry. When considering reconstructive surgery, we
need to make that decision for and about ourselves, not for
or about the men (or anyone else) in our lives.

*Since I am the one with the missing breasts, my
decisions about reconstruction are up to me.*

Seek not to imitate, but to improve, even to perfection,
the excellences of thy nature.

—*Sydney Owenson Morgan*

~

Even my mother has said to me, "Have you considered re-construction?" But the answer is no. I don't want any more cuts, any more anything done to this area other than for it to heal. I like my body better since the mastectomy. I truly believe that I can wear my mastectomy unadorned and still be very pretty.

*It is not how I am, but accepting myself the way I am,
that is essential.*

Nothing is so good as it seems beforehand.
—*George Eliot*

❧

Our task seems overwhelming if we define it as the need to create a sense of physical and emotional symmetry in a world populated by seemingly perfect women and men. But that is not the task. Our task is simply to recollect that there is no perfect symmetry in nature.

Perfection in life comes from living despite it all.

You have to accept whatever comes and the only important
thing is that you meet it with courage. . . .

—*Eleanor Roosevelt*

∾

When I look in the mirror, I am not repelled by myself. I
feel that as a woman, I can absorb this loss. Just be a little
different. I've always liked being a little different. Actually,
I feel exceptional. Having breast cancer and ending up with
one breast is only one of the dramatic things that have happened in my life. And whatever it has been, I've always
turned it into a feeling of being exceptional. I am a person
who doesn't need another breast. All I need is courage.

*Whether I place an implant under my skin, a prosthesis into a bra,
or do absolutely nothing, all I really need is courage.*

And it's often only that they're great sponges. . . .
—*Zoe Akins*

I already hated my prosthesis because it was so heavy. As soon as I got home every day I took it off. Then, the first time I went for a swim, I found out that the fabric around the prosthesis absorbed water. It kind of dragged on one side and I literally had to haul it out and squeeze the water out. It would have been more proper to run off and wring this thing out, but instead I did it right there at the pool. I'm sure it looked as though I was twisting my breast off, but I didn't want the dampness to chafe my skin. I was being defiant. I was angry that this false thing on my body was such a nuisance, but more than that, I was angry that it was there in the first place.

Prostheses are like sponges, very adept at absorbing our feelings—positive or negative—about having to wear them in the first place.

Forgetting a Prosthesis

Mental health, like dandruff, crops up when
you least expect it.
—*Robin Worthington*

❧

I was sailing in rough water, in heavy weather gear with a
T-shirt on underneath. As we got closer to shore, the
weather warmed and I stripped down to my T-shirt. Then
we docked. I jumped off the boat, and went about my business. I tied up, hosed down the boat, and put away the
sails, along with everyone else. It wasn't until much later that
I realized that I wasn't wearing my prosthesis. To my amaze-
ment, I wasn't horrified. At my age, most people are not
looking at my body. But oddly enough, that was still my
hope. To this day I wonder if anybody noticed.

*Celebrate those days when even the most self-conscious
among us forget.*

... Bring me the latest novelties ... [but] if it is only as
good as those which I see other people wear,
I had rather be without it!
—*Isabella D'Este*

∽

I went to a fantasy lingerie shop and put on a merry widow
with garters. I thought maybe I could find someplace inside
it where I could stuff my prosthesis. So I stuffed it in and
bent over, and the prosthesis fell out. I didn't know if I
should laugh or cry, but of course I cried. It's ironic that lingerie, the one thing you might want to use when you
haven't had reconstructive surgery, ends up being almost
as difficult as the experience of shopping for it.

For me, living with a prosthesis is an emotional experience.

Acceptance

Through spontaneity we are reformed into ourselves.
—*Viola Spolin*

∾

I came out of the shower and started to dress. Classical music was playing on the stereo and the kids were out back in the garden. I thought how beautiful the moment was, the music and the voices of the kids, the sun and shade playing on the leaves outside the window. I just wanted to savor it, to soak it in a moment longer, so I put on a robe and stood in the back doorway to watch the kids. They were playing catch.

"Hey, what are ya doing?" I called to them. "Can I play?" "OK," one yelled, and then "Here, catch," and he lobbed the ball at me. I caught it. But what he hurled at me was none other than my prosthesis. They were playing catch with it! Suddenly I knew that the kids had accepted that I wore a prosthesis. And their acceptance made it all the more acceptable to me.

When the child within me reaches out to play, I never know what kind of insight I might catch in my outstretched hand.

Sorrow was like the wind. It came in gusts, shaking
the woman. She braced herself.

—*Marjorie Kinnan Rawlings*

It was three months after my mastectomy when I ambled
in for reconstructive surgery. I looked at all the outstretched
patients on gurneys from the point of view of the well and
the healthy, and I was flooded by sorrow. Did I really want
more surgery even if it was to rebuild my breast? All of the
memories of mastectomy and hospitalization flooded back
and I found myself caught in a kind of resonating fear. I
came in for what I thought of as a positive form of surgery,
but found myself unprepared.

*I acknowledge that reconstructive surgery brings with it
its own set of associations and fears.*

The engineering is secondary to the vision.
—*Cynthia Ozick*

I saw reconstructive surgery as a way of marking the end of this phase of my life. To me, as long as I had only one breast and a prosthesis, it was as though I still had cancer. Reconstruction is a way of ending this particular chapter. Plainly and simply, I opted for reconstruction as a way of leaving the cancer behind.

Reconstruction completes my vision of myself as a healthy and active woman.

You do this to a woman? I dread more
the affront than the pain.

—Maria Cazalla

$\sim$

I had a series of reconstructive operations, most of which
didn't work. I developed a staph infection and I was back
in the hospital for another three weeks. Then I had three
more operations in the course of three years. The ups and
downs of reconstruction are an ongoing process. It isn't
necessarily that you have immediate results. There are problems and risks. In my case, reconstruction followed me
around for a long, long time.

I accept the risks as well as the benefits of reconstructive surgery.

Implants

There must be acceptance and the knowledge that sorrow
fully accepted brings its own gifts . . . It can be
transmitted into wisdom.

—*Pearl S. Buck*

$\sim$

My new breast is a nice little one. It was supposed to look
like a teardrop or a croissant, like my natural breast, but it
ended up looking like a grapefruit. Frankly, I don't care
what kind of breakfast food it is, as long as I have it under
my skin. It fills out my bra without me having to think
about it, and on a basic level, it gets the job done.

> *I'll like my result much better if I don't expect
> another breast from God.*

. . . Sometimes it's a friendly enough curiosity, sometimes
sly and malicious, but you feel as if you were
being eaten alive by fishes.

—*Katherine Anne Porter*

People are curious. They want to see, to touch it. But I
don't like being the object of curiosity. I'm not a freak in
a sideshow. So if a woman asks me if she can see and touch
my reconstructed breast, I tell her sure, as long as I can see
and touch one of her two natural ones.

*Some women gain validation by exposing their new breasts
to others; some women gain validation by saying no.*

Imbalance

When we begin to take our failures nonseriously, it means
we are ceasing to be afraid of them. It is of immense
importance to learn to laugh at ourselves.

—*Katherine Mansfield*

What strikes me funniest about the physical imbalance of my
reconstruction is the idea of it. I can now safely say that I
am the only woman I know with a 50-year-old boob on
one side and one that is only 3 years old on the other. It's
a way of saying that they don't quite match, that they're
not quite in sync—yet they're both mine and I love them.

*When you average in a sense of humor along with the altered
breasts, you can always find something to smile about.*

Disappointment

I was very disappointed by my reconstruction. Despite all the warnings, I expected too much. I hoped that the operation would get me back to being natural looking. But when it was done, I realized that I wasn't anywhere near looking the same and that I was never going to be. I hoped that reconstruction would be the entire solution and that I would have no responsibility in the matter. But I was wrong. Reconstruction is the groundwork for rebuilding self-image, but it does not do it all alone.

*Reconstruction is a beginning point, not an end, in
the process of adjustment to my new body.*

I am no longer what I was. I will remain what I became.
—*Coco Chanel*

∾

I had to massage my new breast morning and night to keep scar tissue from forming and causing my breast to harden. At first I resented it. I wanted my breasts to just "be." I didn't want to have to work at having a breast. I didn't want the constant reminder that there was this foreign object living under my skin.

To my surprise, the daily massage caused a kind of bonding to take place. It helped me to get to know and accept my breast. I learned the limits of my sensitivity—the beginning and end points of feeling at the perimeter of my reconstructed breast and the areas of total numbness. I learned that my breast was made of tough stuff and that I didn't have to be afraid of it. I found out it gets cold to the touch. I felt how when my chest muscles tighten over the implant, massage makes it relax. Most important of all, I learned that my reconstructed breast is a part of me.

I practice daily massage as a way of incorporating my reconstructed breast into my sense of self.

Cleavage

Imagination has always had powers of resurrection
that no science can match.

—*Ingrid Bengis*

It has been nine years of hell and now I finally have had
my reconstruction. Finally! After living for years with an
awful gaping hole, all I wanted was cleavage. Period.

My doctor can't understand it, but what do I care about
a fake nipple to go on a reconstructed breast that nobody
but my husband and I will see? I am a 1950s woman. I
wanted a great cleavage and that's what I got. I think every
woman should be concerned with only those illusions that
mean something to her.

*When I engage a doctor to sculpt my image, I have
him or her do it after my own ideal.*

Nipples

Because God's gifts put man's best dreams to shame. . . .
—*Elizabeth Barrett Browning*

∿

My remaining nipple was going to have to be moved in order to reduce the size of my natural breast. I said to the doctor, "Forget it. What am I going to do with one nipple?" The doctor said, "We can build you another one for the other side." But I said, "No, forget it. I don't want any nipples at all!"

To me, saving my remaining nipple was a nuisance. Once it's moved, sensitivity is reduced. And I didn't want to have to stick wads of cotton on my fake breast to match my nipple in a sweater. I didn't want any nipples. I'm not a young woman. Sex is not that important to me. I wanted the equivalent of two breasts, but I wanted them as simple and easy and as fast as possible.

I do not ask others to justify their choices, nor do I need to justify my own.

As long as I live, I will have control over my being . . .
—*Artemisia Gentileschi*

∽

My reconstructed nipple is kind of like a glass eye. It doesn't do much, just sits there and fills in the blank space so that I don't worry others or myself because something is off, something is missing.

The main advantage of the nipple is that when I'm nude I don't feel like I'm "winking" anymore. My husband always told me that it looked like I was wearing a bra on one side before. I think he feels reassured because there's a focal point for him again. Over and over he's asked me if I'm sure I can't feel anything there where they put the fake nipple. Of course I can't. But we like to pretend that it's real.

The addition of a nipple is icing on the cake, a sense of completion.
It's not really necessary, but if you know you like cake,
why not have the icing too?

However, one cannot put a quart in a pint cup.
—*Charlotte Perkins Gilman*

∼

I am large breasted, and in an ideal world I would want my reconstructed breast to be the same size. But I am unwilling to reduce my one remaining breast in any way for the purposes of reconstruction. I can't see afflicting my one good breast with cuts or changes. I want it preserved as is, a kind of monument to what was.

My breasts are an important part of my sexual pleasure and I refuse to give up my sensitivity. And I plan to have children and breast-feed still, so how can I start reducing and moving things around? To me the functions of my remaining breast—its sensitivity and my ability to breast-feed—far outweigh the visual considerations.

I have considered possibilities for breast-feeding, nipple sensitivity, difficulty of procedure, and recovery time and then the visual, in making my reconstruction choice. I know I'm going to be lopsided and I can live with that.

Matching is important to me, but it is not my primary concern.

The battle to keep up appearances unnecessarily, the mask—
whatever name you give creeping perfectionism—
robs us of our energies.

—*Robin Worthington*

I view my breasts less critically now. Over time, they have become me, despite all their small imperfections. My eye has gotten lazy, casual, just one more glancing observer like any other who might look at them. And if you asked me for an overall impression, I'd say that they are fine, just a part of me, and that I am a woman who is advertising her body still.

Over time, I become less critical of myself.

Implants and Sex

Platonic love is love from the neck up.
—*Thyra Samter Winslow*

∿

I have a friend whom I've known since the age of four. We've both had breast cancer. We've both had reconstruction. She called me up the other night and she kept beating around the bush in her conversation. In a very roundabout way I finally realized she was trying to find out whether it is all right for pressure to be placed on an implant. Finally I just said to her, "Hey, look. If Bob wants to make love to you, go for it. Your implant is like steel. It's going to be OK."

I do not fear bursting my implant in lovemaking—
the plastic is more durable than I am.

... I do not expect or want you to be otherwise than
you are, I love you for the good that is in you,
and look for no change.

—*Mary Anne Lamb*

I think her reconstruction is great. But the fact that there are
scars on her natural breast because she had it reduced affects
me. I don't see what the purpose of those scars is even
though they were voluntary.

On the other hand, I appreciate the addition of a false nipple on her reconstructed breast. I am very impressed by it.
I know it's all cosmetic, like a nice hairdo, but I like to be
fooled. It's a replacement, I know, but if it can look like
the real thing, so much the better. It's kind of like painting
the outside of a house. The outside doesn't make it any
better on the inside, but it's still nice to see it when I come
home.

I accept that I am loved for who I am, with or without
my nipple, with or without my breast.

Relationships

Husbands

It's odd that you can get so anesthetized by your own
pain or your own problem that you don't quite
fully share the hell of someone close to you.

—*Lady Bird Johnson*

My blood tests did not look good and the doctor ordered
a bone scan. I was sure I was dying. When I got home after
the scan, I found my husband jumping up and down on
the lawn. I couldn't understand why he was home, what he
was doing, why he was jumping up and down on the lawn,
waving his arms and yelling. Didn't he know how frightened I was?

It turns out that he couldn't take the uncertainty either.
He went home in the middle of the day and personally
hounded the doctor about the bone scan results. He was
so upset that he began crying over the telephone, and the
doctor was so moved that he made a special effort. Minutes
before I arrived home he had finally called Joe back with the
news that my results were all OK.

There is love implicit in the fact that cancer happens to both of us.

Spousal Support

The reason that husbands and wives do not understand
each other is because they belong to different sexes.

—*Dorothy Dix*

∾

Have you ever listened to two men talk? They talk about
fixing things and doing things. They see the world in an active way. So my husband and I have hit upon a term that
makes a lot of sense to him as a man. He is the subcontractor in my fight with this disease. His duty is to hear me
rage, hear me scream and cry, but he cannot make me well.
I am in charge of that.

*My husband is the "subcontractor" in my fight with
this disease. That makes me the contractor.*

You need that guy like a giraffe needs strep throat.
—*Ann Landers*

∼

The very first thing my doctor said when I opened my eyes was, "Your husband will still love you." His comment was as far away from my fears as could have been. But as it turned out, my husband couldn't handle it.

Within two weeks, he stopped coming home. It was the first time in our 18 years that I ever really needed him, but as I became weaker, he wasn't able to become strong. Coming together after the diagnosis and the mastectomy, we finally both found out who we were. It's an odd thing to say, but if I had not had cancer and had remained married to that man, I would have never become a person. Finding myself divorced following my mastectomy was devastating. But as far as its impact on the rest of my life, I can say now that it was the best thing that ever happened to me.

I recognize that a diagnosis of breast cancer focuses a bright light on all my relationships. I am prepared to handle whatever I see.

Family Disease

A family unity which is only bound together with
a table-cloth is of questionable value.
—*Charlotte Perkins Gilman*

My fantasy was the usual one, the kind that I'm sure every
mother has. I'd be a perfect mother and my husband the
perfect father. My daughter, of course, was to be the perfect child. We turned our lives inside out to have her. Now
it seems so unfair that I end up being a mom who is sick.

One of my toughest realizations has been that if you
have cancer and are a part of a family, then cancer is a family disease. I think about the shaping experience that my
illness has become for my daughter, and the burden on her.
Or how my emotional state affects not only her, but my
husband and the relationship between me and him. Even
though I am the one with cancer, there is no question that
this is my family's disease.

I recognize that what is happening to me affects my whole family.

. . . She wanted a happy world and everyone in it happy, but she was at a loss as to how to accomplish this.

—*Anne Edwards*

My reaction in the aftermath of diagnosis and treatment was to be cheerful. But I also tried to cram all my parenting into two weeks. I wanted to teach my son how to read, how to ride a bicycle, about girls, about clothes, about being a geek or not being a geek, and even where to apply to college. He was only four years old! I have learned to trust that if necessary, he and his dad will figure out some of those issues by themselves. In the meantime, I am here for him. But I have also sent him into therapy. Whatever he is feeling about my battle with cancer, he can't tell me or his father. The best I can do is to give him someone of his own to talk to.

I relinquish the idea that I can protect my child by trying to do it all now.

How true is it, yet how consistent. . . .
—*Fanny Burney*

⁓

The world goes to pieces but some old patterns never change, and sometimes they're a comfort. One woman went to visit her 92-year-old mother at the end of her cycle of chemotherapy treatments. She had only one inch of hair around her head and had put on weight.

"*Who* are we?" the elderly woman asked.

The daughter's heart sank. Was she so changed that her own mother couldn't recognize her?

"It's me," she said, "your daughter!" and took her mother's hand.

"Oh," said the mother sourly. "I liked you better in your wig. And now that it's over, why don't we lose some weight!"

The daughter listened to her mother's critical comments from the bemused distance of a recent bout with breast cancer. It was actually a joy to have her mother back on her case. It was reassuring that despite age, surgery, chemotherapy, and distance, they were both the same two people.

Sometimes it's a comfort that the more things change in our lives, the more our relationships remain the same.

> . . . Think always that, having the child . . . in your arms,
> you have God's blessing there.
>
> —*Elizabeth Clinton*

Chemotherapy has thrown me into menopause. It is not the hot flashes and all the attendant discomfort that I have had to deal with, it is the fundamental loss of my ability to bear children. I am a young married woman and childless, and menopause for me has been like a small death.

But out of that loss and letting go, I have found a sort of rebirth. I have adopted. It is true that because of breast cancer, I have had to let go of what I call my biologic narcissism. I cannot pass on my genetic material. But as a woman who has gone through a year of nausea, I tell myself I don't need another nine months of that anyway. The true impact of being a parent is in raising a child, not bearing one. My parent-child bonds will come from caring for my daughter.

I earn my relationship as a parent by doing it.

Friendship

Best friend, my well-spring in the wilderness . . .
—*George Eliot*

~

It is only very, very good friends that I consent to see in the few days directly after treatment. When you can't trust yourself to be yourself, you need blind faith in the people you have around you. I feel like a wild animal, yet I hope for caring, compassion, and understanding. I want comfort. I want to be an unabashed bumbling idiot yet feel myself still loved.

But the best part of it all, for me, is the relief my friends give my husband. It means that he has more of a life than just being my nursemaid. Our friends' willingness to be with us under these conditions is a show of support. I accept their gift as a wonderful statement of caring.

The caring of friends is a powerful healing tool. I choose that kind of social support for myself.

It is easy to relate what is of no importance.

—*Colette*

I needed to announce the news to others, to say over and over again, "I have breast cancer." It was a way of making the news real. It was a way of integrating this devastating change, this blow to myself. Because suddenly I saw myself as different in relation to others, as though I was marked by cancer and by death. And I imagined that others saw me in the same way. Telling others as randomly and indiscriminately as I did was not necessarily wise, but it was a psychological necessity.

It was a way to construct the reality of the disease. It was a way to dispel the shock and horror and my feelings about myself by driving them out—literally—on my breath.

My need to announce "I have breast cancer" is a way of redefining my relationship to others and of testing if I am still the same person in their eyes.

Pity is the deadliest feeling that can be offered to a woman.
—*Vicki Baum*

∾

News had spread around the movie industry that Jane had breast cancer. "David, why are you here? How's Jane?," someone asked Jane's husband at a party. "She's right here," her husband said, "Ask her yourself." The look on that man's face was one of horror, pity, embarrassment, and shock. He assumed, like most people, that you get a diagnosis of cancer and then you die. It was the first time Jane realized that some people would react that way. But she didn't feel bad about it. She just got pissed off and told him so. "I am the same person I always was," she said.

Rejecting other people's pity confirms my unwillingness to be a victim. I now affirm I am the same person I always was.

May I reach
That purest heaven, to other souls
The cup of strength in some great agony.

—George Eliot

Does it seem easier to you to avoid mentioning breast cancer and its treatments than to face the possible rejection inherent in letting people know? How painful a choice that is, given that your needs for communication and support are now at their greatest.

Reaching out to others is actually a way of working through feelings of self-rejection and alienation. It is an opportunity for those around us to demonstrate their appreciation of us and prove to us, if we need the proving, that we have not changed in their eyes. It is possible to reach out not only to friends, family, and co-workers but to therapists and breast cancer support groups as well. By sharing feelings, we turn the ordeal of breast cancer into an occasion for growth.

By remaining open, I communicate what I need. By communicating what I need, I create the possibility of getting it.

Privacy

While all deception requires secrecy, all secrecy
is not meant to deceive.

—*Sissela Bok*

∼

We may need to resolve our own feelings about breast cancer before we dare risk bringing the news outward and thus
exposing ourselves to the questioning gaze of others. It is
natural to be reticent about ourselves at this time, but pro-
longed reticence may be a signal that we need to examine
our underlying fears.

It is certainly valid to want to look at what the diagnosis of cancer means to us on our own before we share it
with others. It seems a fair decision too, if we wish to share
the news only with our partner or a close friend at first.
Still, we need to examine whether we are consciously or unconsciously locking ourselves away in a prison of silence
in order to sidestep deep-seated fears. The most obvious
fear is that of rejection— the shame-producing expectation
that cancer and its treatment have diminished us in others'
eyes.

*I remember that privacy is a path to adjustment only when it is
born from self-knowledge and not from shame and self-rejection.*

Co-workers

The idea of strictly minding our own business is
moldy rubbish. Who could be so selfish?

—Myrtie Lillian Barker

∽

I never hid from my co-workers the fact of my cancer or
that I was undergoing treatment. That was my choice, my
particular solution. My world had gone crazy, but I needed
to be able to be honest about it. I needed to work and I
didn't want to hide.

There is a benefit in being so forthright. I found out that
everyone I know professionally has had some contact with
breast cancer, either directly or through a friend or a friend
of a friend. I didn't have to feel isolated among them. They
were interested, supportive, concerned. Many were educated
by my experience. They went out and had their own breasts
checked, or urged their wives to do so. My co-workers are
professionals, but they are also human beings.

*My breast cancer experience causes my relationships to grow
and deepen, even my professional ones.*

Life is nothing but a series of crosses for us mothers.
—*Colette*

My children were all grown, but that didn't make any difference. I was worried about them. I worry that they feel
cheated. Or maybe it is me who feels cheated. I want to
share in the joy of their adulthood, having already gone
through the rotten years. I guess the bottom line is that
when it comes to children, we always want to be there for
them a little longer. It doesn't matter how old the children
are—4 or 40—and it doesn't matter how old we are, either.
We always want to just be there.

*No matter how far away or how old they are, today
I tell each of my children that I love them.*

It is not a bad thing that children should occasionally,
and politely, put parents in their place.

—*Colette*

❧

I am a grown woman, but the implicit message from my
parents was, "Take care of yourself and be a good little girl.
Don't die." I know it is hard to see a child sick, no matter
what her age, but I didn't want to be responsible for their
guilt. I find it wonderfully ironic that it wasn't until my
weakest moment that I found the strength to stand up to
my parents for the first time. I didn't want to feel that if I died
it was because I didn't try hard enough, as though I was
doing something bad to them. I was doing the best I could.
It took a life-threatening illness to realize I was good enough
to finally stand up and tell my parents that I was in control.

I love my parents, but I am the one in control of my life.

Quite nice women suddenly have to wear this title with
the stigma on it and a crown of thorns. . . .

—*Sylvia Ashton-Warner*

❧

I attended an extended family gathering. It felt like a gathering for the explicit purpose of staring at *"Mary", who has cancer.* After an hour of it, I think most of them realized it was the same me. I don't think I had any doubts that I was the same me. Let me caution others who go visit distant family or friends: Don't just sit around and "have cancer." Wherever you go, be yourself and have cancer. Then they'll know it's the same you for sure.

*I have a clear message in everything I do. It is that I am
still the same me.*

... To be forsaken and ugly, are the greatest
distresses a woman can have.

—*Elizabeth Inchbald*

~

Just as we are inspired by the degree to which people rallied around us, we can't help but feel abandoned as they fall away. Perhaps we have forgiven those friends and family who, because of their own fears and insecurities, stood at the sidelines. But now we are uncertain if we have the internal resources to also let go of those who have supported us until now. As times goes on, we notice that their visits and calls are becoming fewer and further between.

We feel guilty for our thoughts, guilty about our seemingly bottomless need. But we recognize that others have their own needs, too, even as we acknowledge that our sense of abandonment is real.

*I forgive myself when it feels like others have abandoned me,
but I do not abandon myself.*

I long to speak out the intense inspiration that comes
to me from lives of strong women.

—Ruth Benedict

As women, why struggle on our own when we are part of
a group whose members can imagine how we feel and what
we are going through? Sharing feelings with women family
members and friends is a significant source of support.
Sharing with women who have had breast cancer lends
even more meaning to our experience and purpose to our
struggle. They provide context, understanding, practical
information, and an opportunity for sharing.

Scientific studies prove that support groups have a robust
effect on women with breast cancer. It is a way to curb depression and receive even more specific emotional support
through the difficult process of medical treatments. Turning
to the women around us in all different ways is not just
positive thinking, it is positive action.

I am empowered by the support of strong women.

. . . I cannot deny that, now I am without your company
I feel not only that I am deprived of a very dear sister,
but that I have lost half of myself.

—*Beatrice d'Este*

~

I couldn't imagine why I hadn't heard from my out-of-town sister when I was in the hospital. Finally, after I got home, she called me.

"Where have you been?" I asked.

"In the hospital," she said. "Because of your diagnosis I checked my breasts for the first time, and I found a lump in exactly the same place you did. It was cancer."

My sister had a lumpectomy. I had a mastectomy. My diagnosis may have saved both our lives. It terrifies me that she has breast cancer—since we are both now at greater risk—at the same time that I no longer have to worry about *Why me?*

*I will use my experience with this disease as a caution
to my female family members and friends.*

. . . the silent deep abode of guilt.
—*Mercy Otis Warren*

❧

There is the guilt of being incredibly "lucky" and circumventing treatments that others have not. There is the guilt when a friend or a family member with the same disease does not respond as well to treatment. There is the guilt of simply having survived. How odd that one of the most positive aspects of this experience is the people I encounter along the way. Yet it is exactly because their trials and tribulations so closely mirror my own that makes it all so hard. It is a double-edged sword, this doing well and feeling guilty. Still, I wouldn't have it any other way.

I rechannel feelings of guilt and sadness into positive energy; it is up to me to stand and celebrate life on behalf of myself and others.

··

Concerns of Single Women

I speak what I feel.
—*Marie de Sevigne*

∾

A woman I know was killed in an auto accident a year ago. I was introduced to her husband at a party recently and as soon as I mentioned her name to him he started to cry. My immediate reaction to his tears was to describe my own feelings of loss about the loss of my breast. I wanted to make him feel better, but the more I talked, the more he cried. It was the most awkward moment of my life.

Much to my surprise, he tracked me down a few days later and asked me out. He told me he was very touched that I had responded to his vulnerability with vulnerability of my own. So I learned a lesson. He didn't care that I didn't have a breast, he cared that I had a heart.

The vulnerability I feel as a post-mastectomy woman needn't be a barrier, but a bridge, in all my relationships.

Fear

∾

We had been dating for several months when I found a lump in my breast. What went through my mind was that my life was over. Not just that I was going to die, but that the possibility of a future life with this man was over. It was so ironic. After years of saying that I would never marry again and keeping this man at bay, I was just starting to think that maybe I could spend the rest of my life with him, and then I found the lump. When I found out it was cancer and that my breast was to be removed, I was sure that it was all over between us. I thought that once he knew, he'd be out the door. And when I told him he said, "Oh," and that was all. I thought, well, that's it. No more.

When he stood by during the crisis, I assumed he was just being nice. I fully expected that the romantic aspect of our relationship would never pick up again. So you can imagine my surprise when he proposed to me a few weeks after the surgery and shortly before my chemotherapy treatments began.

Despite my worst fears, a diagnosis of breast cancer may be a catalyst for strengthening my relationships.

> . . . There are times when one is commanded to do
> something even at the price of one's life.
>
> —*Hannah Senesh*

～

I don't know why I deny myself. It isn't like a relationship is something that I don't want and can easily give up. But my feeling has been that for now dating is not possible. If I feel even a hint of interest, it's as though a man is proposing something that is just not possible for me. I simply don't flirt. As soon as I recognize that someone is displaying interest, I avoid him. I have turned off my part of the sexual back-and-forth.

Cancer and mastectomy are difficult enough for me right now without the pressures of dating and the possibility of being sexually active.

I have been sick and I found out, only then,
how lonely I am. Is it too late?
—*Eudora Welty*

∽

The shame that follows a diagnosis of cancer colors our
perceptions of how others see us. Since we are feeling suddenly different, out of control, alienated from our bodies,
and no longer sure of ourselves, we expect that others are
seeing us as less valuable too.

Why jump to imaginary conclusions? Does it make sense
to withdraw on the basis of how we believe others will receive us? Withdrawal assures us of only one thing: isolation. It takes time and practice to discover who we are; the
process, as it docs at any other time in life, means risking vulnerability. But it is never too late.

*I now look inside to see what my feelings of shame have closed off
in me, to figure out how to reopen those parts of myself.*

. . . the strength, the grossness, spirit and gall of choice.
—*Muriel Rukeyser*

～

A man came up to me at church and invited me out for a cup of coffee. I said no. At the time, I thought it wasn't because I was afraid but because I was interested in someone else. But that other person wasn't paying much attention to me. He was safe. He knew that I was having chemotherapy and he was steering clear of me out of fear. I thought about it later on and I thought, *I've got a choice. I've got a guy that's coming up to me and asking me out and I'm saying no. He's enthusiastic and he wants to know me, despite everything that is going on. And I have this other guy that I think I'm interested in and who doesn't give a damn about me, really. So what am I doing?* A week later, I went up to Jerry and told him I was ready for that cup of coffee.

I make use of the new clarity and openness that breast cancer has afforded me in order to make healthy choices.

> The age we call awkward and the
> growing pains it inflicts . . .
>
> —*Colette*

∾

Single women face great emotional risks following treatment for breast cancer. We are like teenagers again, self-conscious and insecure about what we have to offer. At the same time that our self-image and self-esteem have been severely threatened, we face the enormous challenge of laying ourselves open by dating. Like teenage girls on first dates, our questions relate directly to concerns about our desirability, but in this case the questions are "Can anyone tell just by looking at me that I have had a breast removed?" or "Why would anyone want me once they find out I've had breast cancer?"

Recognize that the basic dilemma we face is really the same old Catch-22 of the adolescent dating game; in seeking any new relationship, doubts about self-worth and attractiveness will surface. And just like teenage girls, we feel a sense of accomplishment, validation, and fear when a man reaches out to us in a gesture of interest and acceptance.

I trust that behind my girlish insecurity is the courage, depth,
and wisdom of a powerful woman.

Now suddenly she was somebody, and as imprisoned
in her difference as she had been in her anonymity.

—*Tillie Olsen*

Fear of socializing is fear of rejection, plain and simple.
Beneath the layers of our conscious reasons and excuses
stands a fundamental belief that we are no longer worthy,
attractive, or desirable. We feel we are perpetuating a sham,
passing for normal, when just below the surface is evidence
that we are not.

Cloistering ourselves is a coping device. But by continuing to cut ourselves out of social situations, we run the
risk of eventually undermining, not protecting, our fragile
self-esteem.

Social situations are a testing ground, a way to regain
confidence and experience that, despite our initial fears,
we are not obviously marked by a big C across our forehead
(or our chest). Getting out and about is one important way
to begin rebuilding self-esteem. We need to see ourselves
as we blend in, amuse, attract, and again become the social
and sexual selves we once knew ourselves to be.

*By making social arrangements of all kinds, I resist
becoming a prisoner of my own fear.*

First Date

It is so tempting to try the most difficult thing possible.

—Jennie Jerome Churchill

❧

My first date was a night of approach and avoidance. I felt like a fraud who was passing for normal. I met and conversed with Tom, yet I strained and struggled to end the evening. I came to dine, but I hardly spoke. The effort to suppress the facts of cancer required all my energy. I negotiated my way between his words, looks, and touches very carefully, like an old woman walking downhill on ice.

Now I congratulate myself for those first critical steps. I allowed myself to meet him, to go on the date, and to get through the night. Never mind that I tried to send him away and then had to lasso him back. Never mind that I had a hard time looking him in the eye. Never mind that I seemed to freeze when he touched me. I now count living through all those moments of terror as a major accomplishment, the beginning of the rest of my life.

*I see the emotional risks I take as necessary steps in
my process of positive self-change.*

Sharing

It's astonishing in this world how things don't
turn out at all the way you expect them to!

—*Agatha Christie*

~

I went out all the time. I don't know how I did it. I guess
I never really looked in the mirror very well. But nobody
ever said a word. Nobody ever said that I didn't look well
or that my eyebrows or eyelashes were missing. And whatever I looked like, men still went out with me! I don't
know how they did it. I must have looked bloody awful.
But they were all so nice. And I discovered that because I
opened up and told different men about myself, that they
would open up and tell me some problem of theirs too. It
was an equal exchange of our deepest, darkest secrets that
left each of us feeling mutually accepted.

Even when I doubt myself, I do my best to
trust the best in human nature.

Meeting Men

She did not much like him but she liked his
not knowing her.
—*Joan Didion*

I answered a personal ad as a way of meeting a new man
after my mastectomy and reconstruction. It's difficult enough
to meet men at any time, but more than that, I liked the idea
of anonymity. It meant that we came from two different
worlds, that he didn't know any of my friends and I didn't
know any of his. If things went badly, if I embarrassed myself somehow, nobody would ever know about it unless I
wanted them to. I guess what I was doing was like trying
to rehearse a dance in front of a mirror before going out to
perform publicly. I was finding out who I was again, and I
was looking for a man to practice with.

*When I am ready to date, I will make creative use of
all the resources available to me.*

Now I am beginning to live a little, and feel less
like a sick oyster at low tide.
—*Louisa May Alcott*

On first dates we silently contain our feelings of false wholeness. We learn the value of the attentions of men while
safely upright and clothed. We shift our focus from our lin-
gering doubts about ourselves to savoring a man's appreciation of us. Successful first dates teach us to slay the dragon
of impulse and premature disclosure about what has happened and to control the self-destructive urge for a sexual
encounter for which we are not yet emotionally prepared.
First dates are an opportunity to practice renewed self-
respect, awareness, and control.

My first dates are experiments in how to proceed
with dignity even when I'm fearful.

. . . I learned that true forgiveness includes total acceptance.
And out of acceptance wounds are healed and
happiness is possible again.

—*Catherine Marshall*

∽

We often project onto others what we believe about ourselves. Self-rejection and self-criticism exist within us, yet
we experience them as part of the dangerous landscape outside ourselves.

We expect to be rejected because we have rejected ourselves. Perhaps we have given up because we are demoralized
by the unfairness of what life has dealt us. Why would a man
want us? What do we have to offer now?

We learn to answer such real or implied questions positively as soon as we recognize that what we project into the
world is what we see reflected back. Acceptance from others begins with acceptance of self. Love of others begins
with love of self. New relationships begin, with or without
a breast, with acceptance and love of self.

Before anyone can be there for me, I must be there for myself.

> . . . If you have deceiv'd me as a Friend, I have little
> Reason to trust you as a Lover.
>
> —*Mary Davys*

~

John and Denise had been dating for one year. One night John noticed a book about breast cancer on the nightstand next to Denise's bed. "What's this?" he asked.

"A book for women who have had breast cancer," Denise answered.

"What do you mean?" he asked, shocked. "Have you had it?"

"Yes," she said. She had had a lumpectomy and radiation months before meeting John, but she had failed to mention that fact. And now after a year's worth of opportunities, he didn't ask why she hadn't told him about having had breast cancer before. Nor did she offer any further explanations.

Denise says that after that night she never heard from John again. To this day she is not quite sure why.

I build up trust in order to be honest. I am honest
in order to build up trust.

Doubt indulged soon becomes doubt realized.
—*Frances Ridley Havergal*

~

I had a lot of doubts at first. I thought if some guy is going to lose interest, I want to know before I get involved. So I said something about cancer outright. But that sort of bluntness, when it's driven by self-doubt, is transparent. I wasn't easy about the situation, and that became the problem, although of course I blamed it on having had a mastectomy. Gradually the bluntness subsided. But even after I learned to wait a while, I found that doubt just reared its ugly head in a more subtle way. Because even after a man listened to me and said the equivalent of "OK," I still couldn't trust his acceptance. I found I needed more support than just that. I needed big displays of acceptance. I needed evidence like a love letter or at least an emotional embrace.

I recognize the ways in which doubt colors my perceptions.
But as long as I hold onto that awareness,
I know that doubt will never stop me.

She keeps on being queenly in her own
room with the door shut.
—*Edith Wharton*

What is life but one long risk?
—*Dorothy Canfield Fisher*

∼

Following breast cancer, a single woman may perceive everything as a risk. Every action in the direction of reaching out to others feels like a gamble. "If he doesn't want to see me again, how can I handle it? If I tell him, will he run?"

Instead, begin to view this process as a self-affirming one. We are taking care of the need to grow, change, and chance. We are proving our self-worth and self-respect by being willing to risk. We are confident that if we are disappointed, we will not only survive, but try, try again.

I am getting on with my life, unstopped by the judgments of others.

We can only love what we know. . . .
  —*Anna Letitia Barbauld*

∾

The first man I met was Dan. We had probably been out six times and I did not tell him about my mastectomy. It became more and more apparent to me that I didn't want him to know. "Seeming normal" was the most important thing to me and it caused me tremendous internal conflict, so whenever he tried to touch me, I'd cry.

I suffered all this pain because I couldn't tell. I thought he would reject me and find me ugly and freakish and everything else I was still feeling about myself.

Although it seems the most difficult option, "telling" is often the first step in declaring that we are accepting of ourselves.

... What is human and the same about the males and
females classified as *Homo sapiens* is much
greater than the differences.

—*Estelle R. Ramey*

I enrolled in a woodworking class. The teacher was a lumberjack type named Gus. After the first class, he suggested that we stop and get a beer. After the second class, I sat him down and told him that there was something I had to say. I told him I've had a mastectomy and that I'm very scarred. And he said, "I won't mind your scars if you won't mind mine. But mine are all *inside* me."

*If I don't open myself to the risk of dating and telling, I might
miss some tender human moments when I need them the most.*

It's important to get out of your skin
into somebody else's. . . .

—*Diane Arbus*

❧

After much anxiety, Marcia finally told the man she was dating, a prominent lawyer and an older and wiser man, about her breast cancer and missing breast. "I've had a mastectomy."

"Oh," he answered, surprised. "And I have a small penis."

"Is that a problem?" she asked, perplexed.

"I don't know. Is a mastectomy?" he answered.

Each woman must ask and answer this question for herself. Think how women have heard from men since the beginning of time that our breasts are a part of our beauty. It stands to reason, then, that we will need to hear that we are beautiful without a breast. But how can we even hope that a man will speak that truth until we do? Telling must be the first step in the dialogue. It is an opening to communication.

Communication is the single most important factor in
my emotional adjustment to mastectomy.

You need only claim the events of your life
to make yourself yours.
—*Florida Scott-Maxwell*

~

Sharing news of breast cancer and the physical changes you
have undergone is a moment of great courage and risk. It
is standing up and saying *this is who I am and it is OK,* while
facing the fear of possible rejection.

In the moment that we tell in earnest, we learn something
surprising: The reaction is actually inconsequential. When
we are truly comfortable with ourselves, we experience
only the rush of our own personal power as we tell. True,
it comes against the backdrop of all our struggles to get
there: how we once used verbal aggression, perhaps, trying
to send men away, or how we were once silent, not trusting that anyone could understand.

By deciding to take a true risk, we experience the resolution that has gradually taken place inside us. A day comes
when we are able to courageously announce the news and
hear the response, knowing full well that whatever the reaction, we can handle it.

*Today, I tell, and tell in such a way that I risk
sharing a part of myself.*

Confidence

. . . As awareness increases, the need for personal secrecy
almost proportionally decreases.

—*Charlotte Painter*

After many years as a post-mastectomy single woman, I'm relaxed about telling men about having had breast cancer because I know that if someone can't deal with me, it's fine. I'm not brokenhearted. I have arrived at a strong place emotionally. I have been divorced, married, widowed, and dated all since my diagnosis and mastectomy, and I've come to the conclusion that you can tell a man anything in the world about yourself and if he's the right man, he's still going to be interested in you. If he's not interested, it doesn't make any difference what you tell him. So a woman might as well just be herself. My feeling is that you have to take risks in life or you're not going to get anywhere. Initially, telling a man felt like an enormous risk to me. But the more I did it, the more confident about myself as a single woman, and my worth with or without a breast, I became.

*The man I seek will see me as clearly as I see myself
and will love me for who and what I am.*

Beginnings are apt to be shadowy . . .
—*Rachel Carson*

∽

How do you know when to tell? It should be a rational and considered decision, but also based on intuition. By rational, I mean that I waited to tell him until I was certain I could handle his reaction, good or bad, with my self-esteem and self-respect still intact. That takes a certain amount of planning, awareness, and even self-control. Yet, you have to be prepared for the fact that it can never quite happen exactly when or how you expect. I thought I'd tell him when it looked like we were about to become intimate. But then one day there was exactly the right moment in the conversation, and I realized there was no point in waiting. In fact, I couldn't resist spilling the beans. I was anxious to get it off my chest from the first moment I met him, but I knew that telling him too early would be a big mistake.

The right time to tell is not too early and not too late.
I trust that I will know when it is time.

It is a *moment* that decides the fate of a lover.
—*Hannah Cowley*

The news of cancer and mastectomy is a test. It is a test of our self-esteem, demanding as it does that we stand up with the fact of our disease and the ways in which we feel threatened by it. Our challenge is to overcome fear and recast it into open and straightforward language. Our task is to open up conversation by speaking first and standing witness to the response. But always remember that after we speak, there is another test to be looked after and acknowledged. Telling is not only a measure of the woman, it is also a test of the man.

What I fear as the moment of possible rejection for me is really the moment of truth about him.

I shall drive away my thoughts as soon as they touch upon
dangerous ground. I . . . I shall *deceive myself.*
—*Nelly Ptaschkina*

~

I thought I'd wait until I was on the brink of an intimate
encounter. But I noticed that my secret was starting to in-
terfere with our relationship. By carefully skipping over
the details of cancer and the emotional outcomes of the
disease for three or four dates, it got to be too much of an
omission, a barrier, and a weight. I knew that if I didn't let
down my guard, there wasn't going to be any opportunity
to tell, because the relationship was in jeopardy, at least
from my point of view. It had gotten to the point where I
felt like I was deceiving myself and deceiving him. In an odd
way, I told him because I was trying to save our relationship.

*I recognize that telling is an opening to intimacy, that moment
when privacy gives way to openness.*

Perhaps it is the expediency in the . . . eye that blinds it.
—*Virgilia Peterson*

∾

I was so caught up in my own doubts and insecurities that I failed to allow how he might have insecurities of his own. I foolishly expected a reaction that was black or white, a clear-cut, thumbs-up or -down statement. But all I got back were his fears and doubts, at the same time that he was not rejecting me. I was startled.

I had been nervously anticipating this moment for so long that I thought I had a monopoly on doubt and insecurity regarding dating and breast cancer. But I didn't. Let's face it, he knew even less about it than I did. He was a little bit in shock. I never anticipated the complexity of his reactions, that he might be frightened and at the same time that he would want me to help him master it. All this time I had been looking for some statement about my own value and worth, but it turns out he too had needs of his own.

There are many male reactions to the news of breast cancer, the least of which are a simple "yes" or "no."

... No one is more arrogant toward women, more
aggressive or scornful, than the man who
is anxious about his virility.

—*Simone de Beauvoir*

∾

Joe met me and started courting me in the middle of
chemotherapy, in the middle of my battle with cancer.
You'd think any man who would walk into a life-and-
death situation like that would have to have nerves of steel,
be real macho, sure of himself and in tight control. But
don't look for a macho man at all. Look for just the opposite. It takes a man of feeling.

*The kind of man I seek is the feeling sort who can
offer me the emotional support I need.*

. . . like steel that has been passed through fire, . . . stronger
for having been tested.

—*Elizabeth Duncan Koontz*

When she told me, I did a quick internal check to see if
what she said changed anything. It didn't change anything
for the moment and it didn't change anything for the future. I just filed the news away. She was obviously concerned that she no longer fit the mold of an all-American
female. I understand why it was a concern for her, at the
same time I found it surprising. I thought she was both
wonderful and beautiful, and her news was not an issue for
me.

*I recognize that the issues may be greatest in my own mind, even if
it feels like it is the man who won't be able to handle the news.*

Simple love, with but little knowledge, can do great things.
—*Mechtild von Magdeburg*

∾

When I suggested I might stay over, she got a real serious look on her face and told me that there was something she had to say. I thought, "Oh, my God, she's got children somewhere." What she said was, "I want to tell you I've had breast cancer and had a mastectomy." So I kept waiting. I was waiting to hear the rest of the big news. I thought the mastectomy was the lead into something else, but it wasn't. "Is that it?" I asked her. "Is there anything else you have to say?" "That's it," she told me. "Well, so what?" was my response. I felt as if I had been pushing on a door and suddenly the door let loose and I fell forward. "Hell, I have chronic gas and a fat tummy, is that all?"

I acknowledge that my concerns as a single woman may loom largest in my own mind.

Sexuality

The logic of the heart is absurd.
—*Julie-Jeanne-Eleonore de Lespinasse*

The first time we made love I had on a bra, a blouse, and probably a skirt. I made love with all that on. It was like making love through the little flap in a pair of kid's pajamas. I was so distraught by what had happened to me, I refused to reveal myself. I wanted to make love with a whole body and I didn't consider myself whole. Still, I wanted to make love. What I did was emotionally devastating. Except for the fact that I took my panty hose off, you can say I engaged in fully clothed sex for a long, long time.

In my efforts to prove myself by making love, I pay attention to what about myself I am actually proving.

. . . Those who have taken the terrible risk of intimacy . . .
know life without intimacy to be impossible.

—Carolyn Heilbrun

∾

Intimacy is an emotional and physical closeness that transcends the sexual. Even when it is expressed in sexual terms, it is not limited to the act of intercourse. Massage, hugging, squeezing, kissing, stroking, touching, locking hands, sitting or sleeping together, embracing, and gazing into each other's eyes are also forms of intimacy. But the single most important element in intimacy, sexual or otherwise, is the intimacy of dialogue, the most difficult and potent of all.

After treatment for breast cancer, the chief barriers to intimacy for most women and men are fear and shame. Giving voice to those feelings is the only way for a couple to resolve them. It is important to remember that the ability to share our most vulnerable selves and to ask for what we want or voice what we don't want is at the core of intimate relations between any two people, long married, newly dating, or anywhere in between.

Today I risk sharing my inner self.

I have a woman inside my soul.

—*Yoko Ono*

How can we love ourself or make love when deep down we believe our body has been utterly disfigured and ravaged by this disease and its treatment? There are women who, five years after mastectomy, do not walk around nude or take showers in the presence of their partners, women who make love in a nightgown in order to prohibit all contact with their upper body, including their remaining breast.

Perhaps our body seems ugly to us. Perhaps we have ugly thoughts about it. But only through gradual revelation, testing, and exposure can we change our perceptions about ourself and our body. It is only as we change our thoughts that we change our perceptions. As our body transforms in our mind's eye, the possibility for the slow process of renewed openness returns, and with it, the possibility for true acts of making love.

First and foremost, I love myself.

> Opening the window, I open myself.
> —*Natalya Gorbanevskaya*

≈

My husband has been very affected by the cancer. He has realized that I may not be around, although I plan to be. But because of his sense of loss, his sexual desire has been diminished. Meanwhile I am left to deal with the double whammy of needing more closeness and trying to understand the roots of his physical rejection of me.

I am not an island unto myself, but my husband wants to pretend he is. He hasn't acknowledged that there has been any change, and if I start to talk about it he gets angry. There needs to be more communication between us. I have made efforts, but it is hard to do alone. Now I have taken to putting leaflets around the house that announce post-mastectomy spousal counseling for men. It is clear to me that the men need to talk to each other and get support, just as the women do.

We can only open the window onto ourselves. But in so doing, we open the possibility that others may pass through it too.

The very fact that the . . . soul feels insecure strengthens
its active aspiration to master its insecurity.

—*Helene Deutsch*

~

At first I was willing to make love only as long as he couldn't
see me. I always had a nightgown on, something, anything.
It would slide, pull, move, but as long as I had the feeling
that I had a piece of clothing over me, I felt protected.

More often than not, covering up is our own form of
psychic protection, a coping strategy that sometimes hard-
ens into an unsatisfactory way of life when we find ourselves clinging to a cover-up like a suit of armor, months and
even years later.

It is fair to say that failure "to show," like the failure "to
tell," is a warning sign of an emotional impasse. Each of us
must look at our own insecurities and ask in our heart of
hearts if covering up has gone on too long.

*The solution to my insecurities about my body lies in dealing
with my insecurities, not in covering them up.*

> . . . If you have a body in which you are born to a certain
> amount of pain . . . why should you not, when the
> occasion presents, draw from this same body
> the maximum of pleasure?
>
> —*Isadora Duncan*

As we carry our anxieties and worries about body image
and desirability into the bed with us, remember that our
minds always were and always will be the final arbiter of any
sexual experience. Initially, bittersweet associations are
bound to well up: "My scars can be felt. My chest wall is
numb. I'm out of balance." Stay with these thoughts and
feelings. Cry the inevitable tears that come with the first
experience of an altered body in actual sexual practice.
Encourage your own expectations by gently reminding
yourself that you need and deserve the pleasurable sensations
that are about to follow.

Move from emotional pain into the comfort and luxury
of physical pleasure by putting aside all thoughts and instead letting the impact of the touches build. Receive them
as gestures of pure love, healing, and acceptance.

*I relax into my body and experience it again, as if for the
first time, as an object of beauty and pleasure.*

> . . . a little sunburned by the glare of life.
> —*Elizabeth Barrett Browning*

∼

I had a lumpectomy and radiation. Radiation contributed to the soreness of my nipple and I didn't want it touched for a very long time—I'd say a year. I didn't even want to lean on that side. So I just made a statement to my husband, "Be careful, it's tender." He went out and bought me cotton lingerie because he knew that cotton was all I could stand. That was his way of taking care of me. I suppose it was a little peace offering, a way of saying he hoped that this would enable both of us to feel normal and loved through lovemaking.

I find a way to benefit from feeling normal and loved despite my reactions to treatment.

Are you making love or taking inventory?
        —*Mae West*

∽

There I was, without my hair, without my breast, witho
my eyebrows, without my pubic hair, and still I was desi.
able to him. With his wanting me, I gave myself permissio
to feel just as sexy and turned on as before. If I had to re
sort to a little masquerade, it was worth it.

> *The familiar pleasurable sensations of lovemaking*
> *are a pretty good antidote to almost everything.*

Not always the fanciest cake that's there
Is the best cake to eat!
—*Margaret Sanger*

~

There is definitely sex after chemotherapy if you define sex as including everything you share with your partner. For me intercourse and orgasms became less interesting, and cuddling much more important.

There's how the drugs make you feel, there's the descent into menopause, the loss of your hair, the loss of your breast. How much can you assimilate at once? Without all the rest of it, middle age is challenge enough.

But even with all that, my libido came back. It snuck up on me gradually until I noticed that the engines had started back up. Just listen to your body. It will tell you what it wants from the smorgasbord, whether it's cuddling or intercourse.

*Breast cancer has added to my sex life by making it
more varied and tender than before.*

Be prepared mentally and physically for intercourse
every night this week.

—*Marabel Morgan*

❧

Most people expect that sex during chemotherapy is par-
tially or completely renounced. But what a surprise, that
for some women sexual appetite not only continues but
actually increases. Whatever the complex of psychosocial,
chemical, or hormonal reasons for this, there is a benefit
in knowing it. What better way to shatter the cancer myth
and bring to this illness the possibility of the full spectrum
of human needs and responses even in the midst of treatment?

*It is OK if sex is the least of my concerns; it is OK if sex is a
pressing need. Whatever I feel, I now know I am
not alone in my desires.*

. . . chance, the very worst guardian . . . for . . .
personal comfort.

—*Marguerite Blesington*

∾

My husband is a nice, kind man, but after chemotherapy I
wanted nothing to do with him and I told him so. I left
nothing to chance. I didn't want to share a bed. I wanted
my own physical space. I slept on the couch on the nights
after I had an injection. That way if I wanted to be awake
or asleep, if I didn't want to touch anyone, if I wanted to
lean over into my little bowl next to me, if I wanted peace,
I had it all.

*I hole up under the covers on the couch until I am
ready to be held once again.*

I shall have to conquer myself once
more despite everything.

—*Germaine de Staël*

❧

"I have this friend," Nancy said, "and I remember him telling me, 'Oh, Nan, just think how sensuous it is not to have hair. In fact, I think that when your pubic hair grows back, you should shave it off. That's the way I like my women.' I listened on the phone and laughed. 'No, Michael, I'm going to leave it on when it grows back. It's been missing for quite some time.' 'But how neat it is to be slick!' he told me. And although I just laughed, I have to admit that his insistence gave me a new perspective. It opened me up to the possibility that even this damn pubic hair loss might be erotic. And that new perspective helped a lot with my attitude towards sex and with improving my sense of self."

*I conquer fear and self-consciousness by opening myself
up to the perspective of others.*

This will show your Lordship what a woman can do.
—*Artemisia Gentileschi*

About a month after chemotherapy began, I became very interested in sex. I became the initiator in my marriage, I mean like nonstop, more than I ever have in my life. I am convinced that this new level of desire was caused by the drugs in combination with the fluctuations of my hormones. My sex life was very, very active and very good based on this strong desire. I have never experienced anything like it before or since. It far exceeded anything I have ever experienced before, even the usual peak of libido I used to get around a period.

All I can say is that for about two months our sex life was the best it's ever been and the reason seems to be the drugs. It's odd, but chemotherapy improved my sex life.

I've heard about the other side effects of chemotherapy, but I'll certainly be on the lookout for this one.

Love in chaos did appear. . . .
—*Mary Sidney Wroth*

∽

Sex was my antidote. It was an affirmation of life for me. I was 38 and single with 16 positive lymph nodes, and I flouted most of the unspoken rules that seem to silently govern public conduct of chemotherapy patients. I felt that sex was what I needed and that's what I went out and got. The chemo tired me, but not that much, not enough to stop.

There were times when it was physically painful. My whole body was sore. I bruised. I remember crying and saying it hurt too much because his knee kept hitting my knee. And I looked bloody awful, pallid, sprouty bits of hair. But I needed to be held. And if I had an orgasm, that was an added celebration of life. Basically, even if the doctors had hit me with a locomotive, I would have still sought the company of men.

For some of us, sex is a way to celebrate life, a way to seek reassurance, a way to say, "I'm alive."

. . . I must reluctantly admit that I am not quite as I was. . .
—Eleanor Roosevelt

∼

With the loss of a breast, you mourn the loss of an extremely sensitive erogeneous zone. In very real terms, you miss the lost or altered breast because it was an irreplaceable source of pleasure that is gone or at least no longer the same. It is better to mourn your loss than suppress those feelings.

At the same time that you acknowledge the loss is real, however, don't overlook the possibilities in the present. There are tenderness and value to be found in lovemaking. Do not reject sex out of fear that the experience of it today will fail to conform with all the desires, hopes, and expectations that you carry from the past.

Even in the midst of bittersweet recollections, I enjoy the pleasure my body still affords me.

. . . What's de good of strong arms when de
heart is a coward's?
—*Sarah Josepha Hale*

∼

How do we build a bridge between our altered bodies and
altered self-esteem and the sexual realm? We may feel par-
alyzed by what has been taken from us—ways of being,
doing, and even looking, still fresh in our memory. How do
we bridge the fears and feelings, bury the demons, set aside
the images of what is versus what is gone?

The answer is communication—speaking with courage
and sharing needs. "Don't touch me there just now, it's
too soon." Or, "Please do touch my scar, it needs love
too." Or even, "I feel so ugly," if that is how we feel at
the moment. It is only by expressing such feelings that we
have any hope of receiving the healing warmth of a response, the "You look beautiful to me," that every woman
hopes to and needs to hear.

*Today I share what feels good and right, wrong and not right about
me with my lover.*

The distance is nothing: it is only the
first step that is difficult.

—*Marie Anne du Deffand*

∾

The first couple of months after my mastectomy, my husband said he was afraid of hurting me. But I told him it was OK. Then he said he didn't want to worry, that the worry prevented him from getting sexually turned on. Then he said he was willing to have anal sex, but that was all. Then he started to come home late and fall asleep on the couch. We got so emotionally far apart that making love should not have been an issue at all, but quite frankly, I was always trying to get him to make love to me.

He owned up to it later, that he was trying to get me to leave him so he could be done with the mess. He had married a pretty, perky beauty queen, and by 29 I wasn't too many of those things anymore. But he felt he would be an outcast if he left me. He'd have to live with the guilt. It took me one whole year of my life to realize that no matter what I felt like because of cancer and mastectomy, I didn't deserve the sexual and emotional rejection. I finally gave him what he wanted. I walked out.

Every experience—even the most painful—opens up the potential for change and growth and the movement toward a superior life.

Freedom breeds freedom. Nothing else does.
>*—Anne Roe*

~

There is a good case for why our partner should make the first move. "I have been damaged, my self-image shattered," we say to ourselves. "I need the reassurance of being truly wanted and desired. Without that how can I feel like a desirable woman again?"

But inside his mind and heart, there are also doubts and concerns. "She has been hurt. She is in pain. She is sad. She will tell me when she is ready. I want to be sensitive and not impose myself on her until she is emotionally prepared."

By waiting for him to act, especially when he is waiting for you, you risk feelings of rejection. Assume the responsibility of opening up the dialogue. You are the one who has undergone the change and who knows what you need and when. The way to get the reassurance or caring that you crave is to end the silence.

I break the silence surrounding sexuality and speak of my own wants, fears, and needs.

Anxiety is love's greatest killer, because it is like
the strangle hold of the drowning.

—*Anaïs Nin*

❧

We associate the term *performance anxiety* with a man's struggles to maintain an erect penis. But with worry over the whereabouts of our cover-up if we wear one, whether it is doing its job, or doubts about our desirability and self-image, and our deep-seated fears of rejection, is it possible that we too have developed a kind of performance anxiety?

Just as with the "cure" for the masculine complaint, the very risks we need to take in order to break the cycle of fear that paralyzes us are the risks we fear the most. Ease into them slowly, creating safe boundaries. Perhaps stipulate that intercourse is not the aim. Luxuriate in the immediate pleasure of tactile sensations. Try massage, or gentle touching with feathers or silk, as a way to overcome anxiety about your body and how it looks.

Sensation keeps me in the present moment, far from worry, fear,
and anxiety about how I look.

This is a bond nothing can ever loosen.
What I have lost: what I possess forever.

—*Rachel*

~

My husband is more tender and loving than before. I am
precious to him. We have both seen how easy it is to lose
one another. Yes, breast cancer has taken away my breast
from our lovemaking. But it has added something new. It
has enriched our life together and our love, and conse-
quently, our lovemaking as well.

Today, I acknowledge the bonds that have been strengthened.

You need somebody to love you while you're
looking for someone to love.

—*Shelagh Delaney*

❧

For me, making love with a new man was about testing
my self-image, about putting an end to my crisis of identity. I'm sure it's no different than it might be for a woman
who is forced to begin a new relationship after divorce
or widowhood. There is a transition phase after any life-
altering shock that is initially less about loving someone
else and more about finding ourselves again.

*I acknowledge that sleeping with a new man is, in part,
a search for my own identity.*

Touch

The senses are not discreet!
—*Hannah Green*

I didn't want to deal with it, but he did. So I let him love that side and pet it and kiss it and massage it as a part of our making love. And it has helped break down the barriers. He loves it as he loves me. I used to say that as long as a man loved me for my inside, then my exterior didn't have anything to do with it. But if nobody ever kisses or fondles or caresses my reconstructed breast, then it lacks the attention and love that it deserves. I resisted that idea, but now I've discovered that it is correct. It matters. Having it loved has opened up a lot of emotional doors for me. It's a way of saying, "It's there. It's a part of me. Let's deal with it."

To encourage healing, I share my body physically.

"Living," he had said, "like studying,
needs a little practice."
—*Octavia Waldo*

Since I had never run into mastectomy before, I asked my-self, "Hmmm, I wonder if I am going to have an adverse reaction to this?" I was a little concerned. But my worry about how I would respond was very short-lived. Immediately, I shifted my attention to her. I let her take the lead. I let her show me how she felt at the same time that I didn't steer clear of it. I realized there might be things that she would not want me to do. I expected she would let me know if she didn't want me touching her. But I in-stinctively knew that the side with the missing breast needed attention too.

I acknowledge that sexual uncertainty and insecurity are a part of my partner's concerns, as well as my own.

No rest . . . for the Pilgrim of Love.
—*Amelia Opie*

~

She was the one who always felt badly about not feeling sexual right after a chemotherapy treatment—not me. She had lots of ideas about how much and how often. She worried what I would think, but I didn't think anything. I was experiencing a better sex life than I had experienced in a long time. But I had to tell her once that I didn't want to be *used*. There were times when I was asked or expected to perform when I did not feel like it. So we talked. We had many talks. And to me, the talking was the most beautiful part of our sexual relationship after the diagnosis.

Today I remember that being sexually demanding of others is contrary to the caring and reassurance I seek.

An effective human being is a whole that is greater
than the sum of its parts.

—*Ida P. Rolf*

∽

She was worried about making love until I said to her,
"Everybody knows that airplanes can fly with only one en-
gine." She said that my words were masculine words of
wisdom eminently suited to the occasion. And from there,
we took off into the wild blue yonder of lovemaking without any problems at all.

Here I go into the wild blue yonder.

Meditation

Since everything is in our heads,
we had better not lose them.

—*Coco Chanel*

I am a sexual being. My sexuality is all-pervasive, all-encompassing, limitless. It extends from my head to my toes and from hipbone to hipbone, from cheek to cheek. I am a sexual being up and down my arms and up and down my legs and on my back and shoulders, my neck and my navel. I am a sexual being, and it is obvious in my clothes and in my eyes, in my elbows and in my words, the way in which I carry myself and work and play.

I am a sexual being.

Sex and Nudity

So much of the trouble is because I am a woman.
—Ruth Benedict

❧

Women who are married or unmarried have the same response to nudity the first time around. It's not a function of marital status, but the fact that we are women. It doesn't make any difference if it's our husband, longtime lover, or new lover. It's a question of self-image and body image. Hell, I'm a married woman, my husband has seen me have babies, has gone through labor with me, I've been overweight, he's been overweight and everything else, but still, it was an issue. It's less what he thinks and more what I think. My body has been changed radically and there is sadness. I think whether a woman is married or not, covers herself up or not, has known the man for 20 years or not, that when it comes to the moment of first shared nudity, the sadness is always there.

The sadness I feel about the change to my body unites me with all women who have faced breast cancer.

Realizations

The foolish vanity, whence originates so
many strategems . . .
—*Charlotte Smith*

∾

I had the feeling that my boyfriend was hiding his body
from me, that he was always dressing rapidly after a shower
and never walked around nude. Then one night, he came
into the dining room absolutely naked and sat down and had
dinner in the buff. He proved to me how wrong I was. I
realized that I was the one who was constantly hiding her
body, but that somehow I had turned it all around. I think
it was because I naturally assumed I had already made my
adjustment as a single woman. I had found a boyfriend and
was engaging in an active sex life. It seemed I had made
my way past the big post-mastectomy hurdle. But with
him sitting there nude, I realized that my fear of exposing
myself to him was really the hurdle I still had to cross.

Based on a bond of mutual trust, I face the challenge
of nudity with openness.

Sometimes you wonder how you got on this mountain.
But sometimes you wonder, "How will I get off?"

—*Joan Manley*

≈

Based on my two-breasted experience I was incensed to
think that a man might ignore my missing breast if I exposed
it during lovemaking. Then one day I woke up and realized I never actually risked exposing it. In actual fact, I was
the one who wanted my breasts to be ignored. I was still re-
covering from the surgery and the shock to my self-image
and self-esteem. I covered my missing breast and ignored my
natural one. I can't say what made me finally wake up. I
don't know if I suddenly healed enough to accept my husband's attention or if it was his attention that finally made
me heal enough to notice my own omission. But that's
when I decided it had gotten to be time to completely undress. For those of us who imagined that sex would be the
true act of exposure, a time comes when we realize that
nudity represents a whole other magnitude of risk.

*I welcome change in my feelings and attitudes toward nudity,
a sign of the evolution in my emotional healing.*

To gain that which is worth having, it may be
necessary to lose everything else.
—*Bernadette Devlin*

⁓

What we all need are those rare partners who successfully
recognize and break through the obvious and subtle barriers we erect around ourselves as we attempt to work out our
feelings of self-rejection and the ways in which cancer and
the loss of a breast have changed our lives forever.

If you believe it is a loving man's job to offer gentle,
sensitive, and consistent touch to you, then also acknowledge that it is your job to quell your protests and to receive the healing love—skin to skin—that is being offered
to your wounded self.

It is up to me to curtail the self-rejecting impulse to say "No!"

With what a price we pay for the glory of motherhood. . . .
—*Isadora Duncan*

~

The issue of nudity and sexuality didn't affect me as you might expect, until to my utter disbelief I saw it become an issue with my kids. My two young sons were horrified, utterly outraged, that I might look funny privately, or worse still, publicly, like in a bathing suit. They told me straight off, I had to get another breast and not just a breast, but another nipple so that my two sides would match. Like all kids, they wanted me to be normal and to conform. But more than that, it had something to do with their own burgeoning sexuality. I never would have guessed that my missing breast would cross over to become a sexual issue for them!

Today I recognize that my breasts may become a
sexual issue in ways I never imagined.

There is no creature whose inward being is so strong that
it is not greatly determined by what lies outside it.

—*George Eliot*

∾

I have made a decision for myself. I am willing to let him
touch my scar. I am willing to sleep nude. But I am not
willing to let him see me.

Call it just plain hiding if you like, but I know for myself that this is not just a matter of vanity. Yes, it has to do
with the loss of my breast and my weight gain from
chemotherapy. I'm aware of that, but it's also more.

When I was younger I believed that I had to turn myself inside out for a man. Now I am determined to hold
onto my own special thoughts and feelings. At this stage
in my life, I don't consider myself hiding. I consider myself mature at last and I have come to the conclusion that
I don't have to reveal everything to a man ever again, and
that "everything" includes my body.

Today I examine if I remain hidden out of weakness or strength.

He was not ready to receive what I had to bring.
—*Simone de Beauvoir*

He was a little afraid of seeing my mastectomy. We were in bed when suddenly he turned around and looked me in the eye out of nowhere. It was as though he had been summoning his courage, and finally he said, "I am ready to look."

But I realized that at that moment it was like he was a little kid facing down the biggest roller coaster in the amusement park. He was frightened to death. So I told him no. I had no intention of undressing like that under the circumstances, when I could plainly see that he was just trying to prove himself. For me, the timing was not right.

I need safety to undress and trust my intuition about the right moment for taking that step.

Scars

> . . . To have a crisis, and act upon it, is one thing.
> To dwell in perpetual crisis is another.
>
> —*Barbara Grizzuti Harrison*

~

I was at a group meeting with other post-mastectomy women. One of them mentioned that it was two weeks before she let her husband look at her. My chin almost dropped open. I thought to myself, *only two weeks?*

You see, it took me five years to let my husband look at me again. It was—how shall I say it—self-image. I just felt, *this giant, ugly mastectomy scar. It looks so terrible. Why would my husband want to look at me? It's got to turn him off.* He kept saying, "It's OK." And I kept saying, "Turn the light off." I realize now, so many years later, that it wasn't his problem at all. It was mine.

My scar is a lasting reminder. But hiding it too long from others can keep the pain of it vividly alive long after the scar itself has faded.

> If you were healed of a dreadful wound, you
> did not want to keep the bandage.
>
> —*Ursula Reilly Curtiss*

~

We were in Monterey, away from home in different sur-
roundings. We were going to make love, but I remembered the light was on in the bathroom and as usual I said,
"The light's on. Not while you can see me." This time he
said, "Stop being ridiculous." He exploded, "I want to see
you. I want you to know that I can see you without being
turned off." And suddenly he just took off my nightgown,
he actually pulled it off me after all those years of hiding. I
remember tensing up and my mind racing. But he just went
along. He purposely looked at me and said, "Look, it's light
and you're nude and I'm looking at you. And I want you,"
as if there was no change and no difference.

Finally, it was over, and I just let go. The whole stupid
barrier, the nightgown, the darkness, and that wall that I
had constructed around myself were gone. My other breast
was finally back. For the first time since my mastectomy, I
allowed my husband to touch what was left of me.

I experience nudity as a physical and psychological unveiling.

Emotion constantly finds expression in bodily position.
—*Mabel Elsworth Todd*

∾

Even though I had a lumpectomy, I considered my breast cut off on one side and kind of funny, indented and with a scar. I know it's not as unmistakably altered as with other surgeries, but I felt self-conscious and uncertain about it. So I always made sure the room was dark, and more than that I used body language. If he put his hand on my scarred breast, I'd move away and change position. I'd maneuver. The point is that uncertainty about nudity in a sexual situation also afflicts women like me, women who have had lumpectomies.

My self-consciousness and anxiety about my nude body are valid regardless of the type of surgery I have had.

. . . Avoidance is only a vacuum that something
else must fill. . . .
—*Shirley Hazzard*

❧

While mastectomy made no impact on my continuing to undress in front of my husband or on being nude in bed, I think that my seeming physical openness is misleading. I have been undressing in front of my husband for 20 years, and that part is routine. But the actual act of making love, even though I'm nude, is something else altogether. For now, we both practice avoidance. I don't like being caressed because it feels weird and awkward, and I've told him so. Avoidance is how I've reconciled this feeling of being mutilated, despite the fact that I'm not physically covered up. Based on my experience, I would say that nudity does not a priori mean adjustment.

Nudity is not evidence of my emotional truce with the psychological aftermath of breast cancer, but it is at least a show of my willingness to try.

"I am afraid; I am afraid!" I cried.

"And I too am afraid; but it is better to suffer more and to escape than to suffer less and to remain."

—*Margaret Oliphant*

A woman I talked with told me of how she made passionate love and yet refused to stand up nude in front of the same man not two minutes later. That contradiction, as soon as she admitted it, struck her like a flash, illuminating for her the way in which she was coping. "There is something about standing up before a man apart from the act of making love that strikes fear into the core of me," she said. "I guess I still haven't fully acknowledged that my breast is gone. Sex is one thing, but to be looked at and on display, that is another entirely. I don't know when I'll be ready for that."

Being upright and nude is another emotional barrier I must recognize, confront, and eventually break through.

"You mischievous child!" she cried, in great excitement. "What are you thinking of? Why have you taken everything off? What does it mean?"

"I do not need them," replied the child, and did not look sorry for what she had done.

—*Johanna Spyri*

After you've been pregnant and looked as I have, like a pawnshop symbol with a huge stomach, a smaller breast, and a tiny other reconstructed breast, and after you've given birth with all these people in the room and you look like hell with all this blood and tubes going in or coming out of every orifice, only then do you come to the conclusion, "So what's left to hide?" I'm not self-conscious about being nude anymore.

My self-consciousness limits my feminine identity;
my openness allows me to transcend.

Character contributes to beauty. . . . A mode of conduct, a standard of courage, discipline, fortitude and integrity can do a great deal to make a woman beautiful.

—*Jacqueline Bisset*

～

The physical beauty of a woman has never been limited to the perfection or imperfection of her face or body for me. It's how those two are enlivened by her spirit. So it wasn't hard for me to see Beverly nude or to look at her scars. It's just what those scars represented. They were visual images of a knife cutting through that area. It's made me feel sympathy for the process and for the woman, at the same time that I regarded them and her with awe, as though those scars were a badge of courage.

When I stand in the nude, others see character and courage, both of which make me more beautiful.

The mammary fixation is the most infantile—and most
American—of the sex fetishes.

—*Molly Haskell*

∼

Contrary to popular belief, my idea of a woman's body is
a buffet, a smorgasbord. After her mastectomy, I picked
different things from the smorgasbord, which is exactly
what I would have done anyway. It was what I always did
with any woman. I didn't ignore her breasts, but I didn't
concentrate on them either. As to the reconstructed one,
when she revealed that to me for the first time I found that
to be like an imitation sundae. But lest that sound too harsh,
I want you to know that in the end I married the woman
on the other side of that dyed red cherry sundae.

I accept that despite my doubts, men love the person,
not the breast, even in the nude.

I have a great objection to seeing anyone, particularly
anyone whom I care about, lose his self-control.

—*Eleanor Roosevelt*

∿

She was very interested in my reaction to her mastectomy.
She was beyond talking about it. She wanted to show me.
And looking back now, she was under a lot of emotional
stress, because what she did with me—a virtual stranger at
the time—was inappropriate.

My thoughts were that this was rather odd. What was this
lady doing? I had never been anywhere when the first time
you get together with someone, they take off their clothes.
I was uncomfortable, but not because of the mastectomy.
It was more that I could see that she was slightly out of
control, driven by her psychological need. She needed to
show herself to a man and she needed to get feedback. I
found her urgency a little desperate and disturbing at the
time.

*I forgive myself for the clumsy ways I struggle back
toward a feeling of wholeness.*

What if my words
Were meant for deeds?
—*George Eliot*

When she wore something to cover up, it was like an implicit agreement between us that her chest region was off limits. It was as if we both had decided that we were going to ignore the change that had taken place.

I was relieved when she stopped hiding. It was a step forward. Yet I wanted her to take another. I wanted her to take the lead. I wanted to hear her say, "I want you to touch me there." I wanted her to move my hand there. If she had told me, "Feel me there, kiss me there, do things there," I would have been more certain. Instead, I still relegated her breasts to something somewhat hidden or unimportant, like a shoulder.

It comes down to communication. Her undressing was symbolic, it said that she was ready to be more open. But what that meant practically, just how much touch and attention she wanted or was willing to accept, was something that still needed to be negotiated and discussed.

Unveiling is a symbolic deed, but also a beginning point for words.

How quick come the reasons for approving what we like!
—*Jane Austen*

∽

Joe was in bed and I was in the bathroom brushing my teeth. When I finished I took my clothes off and walked into the bedroom. My mind was a million miles away and I totally forgot that I was stark naked. I just strolled out, and Joe looked up at me in a very peculiar way. He had never seen me nude before. When I realized what I had done, I screamed, "Oh no!" and tried to cover myself as best as I could. But Joe said to me, "What are you doing? Stop hiding. Just come over here."

I went and stood by the bed, and he took a moment or two and he looked at me and at the scar. Then he said, "That really looks OK. Now get in the bed," and that was the end of it. From that moment on, the need to cover up my body was totally over and done with.

Nothing is more healing than acceptance and approval.

A miracle has happened! The light of understanding has
shone upon my little pupil's mind, and behold,
all things are changed!

—*Annie Sullivan*

When I was a child, my uncle lost his leg. I was told I
wasn't supposed to stare, but he had to kick his knee and
kick his foot to make it bend when he sat down. And you
know how it is when you are five years old—you say, "Oh
my," and you go up and play with it. My first reaction was
one of fascination and a sense of its being acceptable because my uncle was still the same person that I had always
known and loved. But my parents kept saying, "Don't
touch." Eventually I learned from that that there is something terrible and forbidden about fakeness on the body.

As a post-mastectomy woman, I have come back around
to my original innocent way of thinking. I've already been
through the cover-up stage, but now I don't feel the need.
It seems silly, because in the end I am going to be naked and
after all, I am still the same person.

As my self-understanding increases, I skip the illusions altogether.

Transformations

Every great mistake has a halfway moment, a split second
when it can be recalled and perhaps remedied.

—*Pearl S. Buck*

There was a ten-ton breast sitting in the middle of my living room. It was going to bed with me at night and following me around everywhere. It was going to consume me
if I didn't get past it. Then came a decisive moment when
I realized I had to move on psychologically and make living with breast cancer an event in my life, rather than the
whole thing.

*Today I'll check to see if anything is sitting in the middle of my
living room and what I can do about it.*

And all that we are sorry for is what we haven't done.
—*Margaret Widdemer*

~

Risks don't look like risks anymore, but like experiences and opportunities for growth. They seem like a gift. "Hey, I can take a risk today," is a wonderful feeling when so recently I feared that I might be cut off from risk—or life, for that matter—altogether. Risks don't seem so hard anymore, next to a measure like that.

But if emotional risk taking is easier, I am also more conservative physically. I want to protect my body, which is the other half of the risk-taking equation. I realize that in order to continue the process of freeing myself emotionally, I need to cautiously preserve my body at the same time.

I guard my body as I open my heart and mind to the world.

I wore out the darkness
until lazy dawn.
—*Izumi Shikibu*

Living with the fear of cancer is a catalyst, an opportunity for reevaluation, insight, and change. This is not to say that we don't also have negative and frightening thoughts and that we aren't sometimes overwhelmed by the fear of recurrence and fear of death. Do we deny them? Do we hold back what we truly feel? The answer, of course, is no. But we transpose the tragedy of what has happened to us into something positive.

Part of the learning experience of cancer is taking permission to stay with what we feel, no matter how ugly. By allowing ourselves to fully experience even our blackest fears, we are trusting that something positive will flow from our descent into the abyss. Just as there can be no shadow without bright light, it is only in facing the darkness within us that the possibility of light and insight eventually emerges.

It is within my power to turn fear into a positive opportunity.

Aches and Pains

Prophecy is difficult, especially of the future.
—*Ancient Chinese proverb*

∾

It's the old story: fear and panic at a new ache or pain, at every sniffle and cold. But these are bound to occur, the same minor ailments that went unnoticed before we had cancer.

Living with cancer means living with vulnerability and fear. But since no one can prophesize the future, take a positive attitude even toward aches and pains. It is important to be vigilant, but also optimistic. While pain may be a sign of something ominous, isn't it possible that life has simply normalized so much that what we're experiencing is just the good old, everyday variety of complaint?

My confidence in my health grows with time. In the meantime,
my attitude is critical to my peace of mind.

... It is the promise of death and the experience of dying,
more than any other force in life, that can
make a human being grow.

—*Elisabeth Kübler-Ross*

I am a little bit hyperkinetic, a little bit anxiety prone, in my daily life. Imagine my surprise when I didn't experience cancer in those terms at all. Quite the opposite. Living with the fear of death has caused all my superficial anxieties to suddenly disappear. I have been calmed by facing cancer and the forces of life and death.

Living life while acknowledging death calms the once-
chaotic surface of my day.

Peace, she supposed, was contingent upon a certain
disposition of the soul, a disposition to receive the gift
that only detachment from self made possible.

—*Elizabeth Goudge*

~

Detachment from the pressure of whether or not we are
doing "well enough" in life is one of the benefits a brush
with cancer provides. We separate ourselves from our need
to strive. We distill where our energies go. This is neither
"copping out" nor selfishness, but *the self* coming to the
fore. Separation from the false urgency of life and a heightened sense of awareness about what is truly meaningful are
among the positive perspectives that a diagnosis of breast
cancer brings.

*The insights that come from detachment provide me
with a new standard by which to live.*

Nobody ever flunked breast cancer.

—*Anonymous*

We want to know if we picked the right options in breast cancer treatment, as though breast cancer was some big math test in the sky. We want to know how we've done. We think, God knows, and we'd know too if only we could sneak a peek at the answers in the back of that big black book.

We want to know in order to return comfortably to an illusion. What we are seeking is a way to reembrace the fantasy that we will live forever. But sooner or later we face the fact that when it comes to life, there is no single and certain right answer except the acceptance of uncertainty.

The only certainty there is in life is what I discover about myself in the process of living it.

. . . That is what learning is. You suddenly understand
something you've understood all your life,
but in a new way.

—*Doris Lessing*

∽

I attended a ballet recital. All I could see were the hands
of the dancers, the bowed arms and the graceful hands.
That's sort of unusual, wouldn't you agree? After all, what
do you think when someone says "ballet"? You think of
feet and toes and legs and leaps. I had a vision of myself as
the only person in the entire audience who was focused
on the fingers and hands of the dancers.

Later that night I couldn't sleep. I wrote a poem about
that moment in the ballet that says a whole lot more about
the cancer experience than anything else. Noticing hands
at a ballet is a metaphor for the fact that cancer opens our
eyes to more than the obvious in life. I realized that I was
looking at the world in a new way.

*The transformative experience of cancer has made
every experience fresh.*

The past was nothing to her; offered no lesson which she
was willing to heed. The future was a mystery which
she never attempted to penetrate. The present
alone was significant. . . .

—*Kate Chopin*

The challenge of any cancer is knowing that we might die.
We have always known it, but now we are experiencing it
in a new way. It is no longer an abstraction. The fear trembles
through us, wells up, engulfs us, reduces us to cries,
screams, wails. It is so damned unfair!

The first challenge, the one that has consumed us until
now, is to know that naked fear. The second, which consumes
us at this crossroads, is to know fear and yet to begin
to recognize the gift in it—the gift of the present moment.

*I now live with a heightened appreciation of each
present moment in life.*

O the green things growing, the green things growing,
The faint sweet smell of the green things growing!
—Dinah Mulock Craik

❧

Imagine a beautiful garden, with flowers and plants and 12 million leaves. One day we go into our garden and see that there is blight on a dozen of the leaves. So we kill the blight. Maybe the blight later comes back, but still the garden as a whole is every bit as wonderful as it was before.

Living with cancer is like living in a garden of 11,999,988 beautiful leaves out of 12 million.

I now concentrate on the thriving parts of me.

Faith

When nothing is sure, everything is possible.
—*Margaret Drabble*

∾

I believe that things are meant to be. I hold that belief, but not in any negative sense. I believe that whatever is handed to me, God and I—that great spirit that we each call by our own name—will handle it.

Make peace with whatever comes. I have made peace with the fact that not everyone lives to be 80. I have made peace with the fact that I can't always be with my family and friends. Even if I stick around, they might not stick around for me. I have made peace with the fact that nothing in the world is forever. Nothing stands still. We have to let go of our possessiveness.

Faith is the ability to know death and still go on with life.

Benefits

Throughout my life, I have always found that events which seemed at the time disastrous ultimately developed into positive blessings. In fact, I have never known one instance when this has not proved to be the case.

—*Elisabeth Marbury*

Is it really turning things around too much to consider ourselves one of the lucky ones in life, in that we have already been face to face with what most others hope never to meet? It is not what we would willingly choose, perhaps, but having been through it and handled it, aren't there countless benefits?

Aren't we stronger? Isn't life more precious? Isn't there a new fearlessness? Isn't there a new clarity? Don't we know, deep down, that we have been given an unusual opportunity? The list goes on and on.

Today, I count my blessings.

In order to be irreplaceable one must always be different.
—*Coco Chanel*

Cancer has strengthened my relationship with my husband and has brought us closer together. Just two weeks after I had my breast surgery, my husband had a hernia operation. We shared naps and pain pills. Then one day, literally, a light bulb went out. I climbed up the ladder to try to fix it, but I couldn't lift my arms. My husband could lift his arms, but he couldn't get up the ladder.

When that light bulb went out, another light bulb—the one in my head—went on. We are everything to each other. We're all that there is in this life—our partnership, like two halves struggling to keep ourselves in the light.

*I acknowledge my connectedness to those around me
and to all living things.*

There are no sick people in North Oxford. They are either
dead or alive. It's sometimes difficult to tell
the difference, that's all.

—*Barbara Pym*

Now that we can tell the difference between what is dead
and alive in our own lives, how can we afford to let fear par-
alyze and destroy our today? Isn't there something else more
precious to focus on? Take in all the bittersweet beauty of
being alive. Find indescribable pleasure in the smallest things,
even the way the sunlight falls on the sidewalk and how
the warmth of the sun feels on our hands. Yes, the cliches
are all absolutely true. In facing death, we finally have the
opportunity to savor life.

From inside fear, I discover that the world is even more beautiful.

Some things are very important and some are very
unimportant. To know the difference is what
we are given life to find out.

—*Anna F. Trevisan*

~

I have a tough new reference point for all things, the kind
of scale where most things don't measure up. I may not
get that promotion. Fine. If I don't, I'll stay in my current
job and enjoy my time taking classes. What an easy win.

Some jerk cuts me off on the road. Fine. Let him get
there first, poor fool. It's not life or death, so who cares?

My new internal reference point has put an end to negative cycles. Because for every situation, there is the silently
articulated question, "In the scope of life, is this worth it?"
I ask it all the time and the answer is usually no.

Life is better with my internal thermometer reset.

The world is quite right. It does not have to be consistent.
—*Charlotte Perkins Gilman*

~

Just as life is part of life and death is part of life, the over-all experience of cancer embraces both death and a kind of emotional rebirth simultaneously. To seem to die and then be born all at the same time is one of the paradoxes of a diagnosis. But then, life itself is a paradox, seeming as it does to hold a past and a future in what really only ever is the present.

I accept the wisdom of paradoxes.

People change and forget to tell each other.
—*Lillian Hellman*

∿

I have changed. I now see each moment as urgent. I now see how each moment holds a risk, and I welcome the opportunity to take them because the experience of cancer demands that I live honestly. Cancer demands that I be open. Coming out the other end of this, I discovered that I am not interested in smoothness and acceptance unless acceptance comes from being honest and being myself.

I now make my feelings clear.

Opportunity

It's them as take advantage that get advantage i' this world.

—*George Eliot*

⁓

How does a major illness transform itself from a tragedy into an advantage?

It starts with the keen sense of appreciation of life. It deepens into a release—a letting go, not of life, but of all the petty annoyances that once clouded our perspective of the transitory nature of things. As the importance of things recedes, the importance of relationships comes to the fore and we set about them with a heightened intensity. We really have them. We know what we feel and we say what we think. We know what it is we wish to accomplish. There are pain and joy in equal mixture in every moment, and ironically, we feel ourselves more alive than ever before. We have found a new way of being in the present.

I am transformed by the opportunity to find out who I really am.

My darkness has been filled with the light of intelligence,
and behold, the outer day-light world was stumbling
and groping in social blindness.

—*Helen Keller*

Getting on with life is not blindly charging ahead. It is
asking what do we really want out of life and what is important? If we let life go on unexamined once treatment has
ended, we miss the meaning and the opportunity in suf-
fering, sacrifice, and pain. Dignify your experience by
opening your eyes to its lessons and applying them at every
turn.

Breast cancer is a hard-won lesson in learning how to see.

Don't be afraid that your life will end; be afraid
that it will never begin.

—*Grace Hansen*

∾

It took the threat of death for me to actually live.
1. I was lackadaisical.
2. I was a real worrier.
3. I rehashed the past.
4. I bought clothes and then saved them,
   clothes that I had never worn.
5. I let other people rule my life.
6. I was a doormat.

I feel like I've been liberated.
1. I empathize and sympathize with people now.
2. People are important to me.
3. I am more open and so are they.
4. I can see who really hurts.
5. I feel for people and things.
6. I am not passive.
7. I have conflicts.
8. I am willing to fight.
9. I have developed an inner voice.

*Today I make a laundry list of how the threat of death finally
woke me up and how, in many ways, it is the best
thing that ever happened to me.*

Houses are like the hearts of men,
I think;
They must have life within. . . .

—*Leonora Speyer*

❧

Something shifted inside when I was diagnosed. I truly invested myself in people and human relationships, rather than anything permanent. Screw the house and the garden. People were suddenly so much more important.

When I look at where I am today, I am grateful not for what I own, but for who I am with.

. . . We could never learn to be brave and patient,
if there were only joy in the world.

—*Helen Keller*

Breast cancer is nothing if not a training ground for learning to overcome fears, barriers, obstacles, and insecurities, one after another, learning to find my way over, under, or around them. Some obstacles simply evaporate in the face of cancer. Others, I mastered because of the urgency that cancer brought into my life. It's not that the fear goes away. But by now I am actually skilled at knowing how to overcome feelings of fear and helplessness. I am like some medieval warrior with my lance tilted, ever ready should new challenges present themselves.

Meeting the challenge of cancer has strengthened my sense of self.

The fears of what may come to pass,
I cast them all away,
Among the clover scented grass,
Among the new-mown hay.

—*Louise Imogen Guiney*

The fears of recurrence are the fears we have already faced: fear of pain, death, and debilitation. Since we have faced those fears once and have kept hope alive, we are already seasoned experts at what we need to continue to do. The worry over whether we have a future and for how long runs the risk of poisoning the present moment. Focus on today instead of the future, and keep today from being a mess of sodden sadness. Dig into the everyday and be thankful that today you wrote a poem or saw a friend or did the laundry or picked up your kid at school.

I have the power to make this day a good one.

I live in the ever-present now.
—*Jane Gibbons-Knopf*

≈

There is no word in the Hopi language for past or *future*. There is only *becoming*. If we stay where we are, in the ever-present now, we can't be overwhelmed.

When it comes to living day by day, I only speak Hopi.

I used to trouble what life was for—now being
alive seems sufficient reason.

—*Joanna Field*

∾

"What's happening in your life?"
"I'm alive!"

When people ask me what's happening in my life,
"I'm alive" is what I answer.

Index

Abandonment, 65, 174
Acceptance, 137, 239
Aches and Pains, 259
Active Patient, 73
Adjustment, 140
Adolescent Feelings, 115
Adoption, 162
Advice, 130
Affirmation, 128
Alienation, 52
Alive, 280
Anesthesia, 50
Anger, 10, 71, 116
  Turning into Action, 88
Antidote, 221
Avoidance, 246
Awareness, 263

Benefits, 267
Betrayal, 192
Bucking the System, 29
Burden of Secrecy, 202

Calm, 260
Certainty, 30
Challenge, 277
Checkups, 104
Chemotherapy
  First Cycle of, 74
  Motherhood and, 97
Choices, 25, 184
Cleavage, 148
Closure, 139
Clothing, 55
Commitment, 69
Communication, 38, 197, 223
  Opening up, 211
Completion, 150

Confidence, 199
Conflicting Emotions, 208
Conflicting Opinions, 33
Confrontation, 109
Contemplation, 56
Continuity, 121, 161
Control, 18, 54
Coping
  Qualifications for, 20
  with Blood Counts, 89
Courage, 6, 133, 198
Co-workers, 170
Criticalness, 152
Cumulative Effects, 90

Dating with Dignity, 190
Death Sentence, 7
Deciding, 36
Decision, 41
Delayed Diagnosis, 8
Denial, 114
Depression, 79
  Post-Treatment, 103
Detachment, 261
Disappointment, 146
Discovery, 253
Doubt, 193
Drains, 58

Elective Surgery, 138
Emotional Chaos, 14
Energy, 86
Exercise, 81, 123
Exhaustion, 111
Expectations, 222
Exposure, 238
Extended Family, 173

Faith, 68, 266
Family Disease, 159

Fear, 112, 181, 258
  Middle-of-the-Night, 98
  of Being Wrong, 34
  of Death, 269
  of Recurrence, 91
  of Treatment, 44
Feedback, 125
First Date, 187
First Lovemaking, 213
Flux, 35
Friendship, 163
Future, 278

Get It on Tape, 28
Giving Yourself Permission, 92
Goals, 95
Grief, 13
Grown Kids, 171
Guilt in Relation to Others, 177

Hair Loss, 82
Hiding, 113
Honesty, 272
Hope, 83
Humor, 48, 87
Husbands, 156

Imbalance, 145
Implants, 143
  and Sex, 153
Indecision, 22
Infatuation, 126
Information Control, 24
Information Gathering, 23
Initiation, 225
Insecurity, 203, 212
Insight, 274
Intention, 127
Interference, 39

Internal Conflict, 45
Intimacy, 209
Isolation, 16, 64

Joy, 122

Leaving the Hospital, 63
Like a Teenager, 185
Living
  in the Present, 264
  Life, 275
  with Cancer, 265
Loss of Pubic Hair, 219
Loss of Self, 19
Love, 124

Male Perspective, 154, 205, 206, 230, 231, 232, 249, 250, 251, 252
Man of Feeling, A , 204
Massage, 147
Mastering the Confusion, 26
Matching Breasts, 151
Meditation, 40, 233
Meeting Men, 189
Memory Loss, 100
Menopause, 85
Mirror Gazing, 110
Moment of Truth, 201
Morning After, The, 51
Mourning, 107
Moving On, 256
Myths, 217

Newly Single, 158
Nipples, 149
Nudity, 236
  and Family, 240
  and Lumpectomy, 245

On Display, 247
Openness, 248
Operating Room, 49
Opportunity, 273

Pain Medication, 53
Paradoxes, 271
Parenting, 160
Parents, 172
Partnership, 268
Pathology Report, 61
  Waiting for the, 60
Perfection, 132
Performance Anxiety, 226
Personal Comfort, 218
Pity, 165
Politeness, 96
Prayer, 84
Preciousness, 227
Preparing for Treatment, 75
Privacy, 167
Private Partings, 46
Process, 108
Prosthesis
  Discomfort, 134
  Forgetting a, 135
  Shopping and, 136

Rage, 11
Rape, 106
Reaching Out, 166
Realizations, 237
Receiving Treatment, 76
Reference Point, 270
Relaxation and Treatment, 77
Release, 244
Remaining Hidden, 241
Resentment, 118
Respect, 37
Restlessness and Irritability, 99
Results, 141
Right to Choose, The, 31
Risk Taking, 194, 257
Risks, 142

Scalp Treatment, 80
Scars, 243
Self-Acceptance, 131, 191
Self-Blame, 17

Self-Image, 119
Self-Involvement, 228
Self-Love, 117, 210
Sensitivity, 214
Sex and Chemotherapy, 215
Sexual Rejection, 224
Shame, 183
Shared Effort, 72
Shared Farewell, 47
Sharing, 188, 216
Shock, 9
Sisterhood, 169
Sisters, 176
Social Life, 94, 186
Spousal Support, 157
Statistics, 32
Support Groups, 168

Telling, 196
  Not Telling, 195
  Telling Others, 164
  When to Tell, 200
Terror, 12
Timing, 242
Today, 279
Touch, 229
Transition Time, 59
Travel, 93
Triumph, 102
Trusting Yourself, 27

Uncertainty, 262
Understanding, 254
Unwanted Curiosity, 144

Validation, 120
Values, 276
Visualization, 70
Vulnerability, 78, 180

Walking the Corridors, 57
Wave of Desire, 220
Weakness, 62
Withdrawal, 182
Women, 175
Work, 101
Working Through, 15